FUNCTIONAL DENTAL MEDICINE

Praise for Dr. Michael Gelb and *Functional Dental Medicine*

Dr. Michael Gelb, like his father Dr. Harold Gelb, is a true visionary and pioneer! Their collective contributions to the health care professions have served to elevate and restore dentistry to its proper role as an integral and vital part of medicine and healthcare. With this book, Functional Dental Medicine, *including his concept of AirwayCentric® dentistry, Dr. Michael Gelb explains how maintaining a healthy mouth will greatly reduce our risks for heart attack, stroke, cancer, dementia, and other chronic diseases. Anyone committed to restoring the health of themselves and their loved ones needs to read, understand, and follow the simple message contained in this book.*

—Richard D. Fischer, DDS, ND, FAGD, FAAO, MIAOMT

Diplomate, ABDSM

Like the inside of your mouth, this book is fresh and clean. Dr. Gelb's new book is innovative and thought-provoking. For the first time a dentist looks at the whole person, connecting how we breathe to the bacteria we house in our mouth. As he says, Dr. Gelb is not a "fill, drill, and bill" kind of dentist. The connection between mouth bacteria and chronic inflammation of the body needs to be heard. Dr. Gelb's words and contribution to dentistry are beyond reproach.

—Patrick Fratellone, MD

Cardiologist, herbalist, and author

Functional Dental Medicine *is a very timely and important book. As a functional medicine doctor, I rely on a team of different practitioners to address the multitude of symptoms when treating and preventing chronic illness in patients. Dentistry is so often put aside by medical doctors, but as we see here in this book, it should be first-line therapy in treating and, more importantly, preventing chronic disease! Collaboration cures, and I am proud of my associations with like-minded dentists such as Dr. Gelb. Together we can make huge impacts in healthcare.*

—Dana G. Cohen, MD

Medical Director, Complete Wellness

Coauthor of Quench

Dr. Gelb's book is a perfect example of where the profession of dentistry needs to go, and he's already there! A properly trained dentist can recognize sleep disordered breathing issues—such as obstructive sleep apnea—decades before a medical doctor recognizes the symptoms. Gelb writes eloquently about how this early screening is possible and about the unique position dentists are in due to their training and knowledge. He not only provides solutions and actionable steps that a patient can take, but also gives them hope long after conventional medicine has failed them. This book is not just for the layperson; I encourage all dentists to read this book A.S.A.P., as it's up to our profession to weigh in on this world-wide epidemic that needs to be addressed with the utmost care and detail. Dentistry is poised to be a major contributor to the solution, and Dr. Gelb is one of its practitioners that is leading the charge.

—Daffnee Cohen

Online marketing expert

DR. GELB'S

FUNCTIONAL DENTAL MEDICINE

How Complete Health Dentistry
is ***Revolutionizing America***

MICHAEL L. GELB, DDS, MS

WITH: **Charles Whitney**, M.D.
Gina L. Pritchard, MSN, RN, CNS, ACNP, DNPc

THE COMPLETE HEALTH PRACTICE SERIES

Printed in the United States of America.

CONTENTS

CHAPTER 1

MAKING A DIFFERENCE

As humans, we need to breathe—that's essential. Especially during sleep, having an open airway is crucial to getting a sufficient amount of oxygen to ensure our bodies stay healthy.

Today, the dental team is perhaps the best healthcare specialty to manage the airway. We're in a great position to identify problems first because we work inside the mouth all day long—we work with the tongue, the soft palate, the upper and lower jaws. And the mouth is one of the key places in the body to address issues with the airway. The airway determines how well you breathe and is governed by your upper and lower jaws, your neck, and your nose. Your airway can be changed by doing simple things such as improving your posture, or it may require somewhat more aggressive treatment such as correcting a deviated septum or removing obstructions in your nasal passages. One of the key things that can change an airway for life is to use an expander on a child as young as four years old.

The airway is an area of dentistry in which I've practiced my entire career—even before I became a dentist, I understood the importance of the airway. You see, my father, Harold Gelb, DDS, was a pioneer in disorders of the temporomandibular joint (the jaw joints), commonly known as TMJ. He wrote the groundbreaking book *Killing Pain without Prescription*, in which he shared insights unknown at the time about how the body systems are connected and how many problems start in the mouth. When I was a teen, I spent a lot of time at my dad's office, looking at the slides he used for his lectures and talking with patients and hearing their stories of hope and how their pain had been alleviated and their lives restored. Many of them told me how their headache and jaw pain, neckaches, and ringing in the ears had been alleviated and how they were really able to enjoy a fruitful and pain-free, successful life.

He also had other providers in this practice: a nutritionist, physical therapist, and biofeedback technician, so I was exposed at a very young age to a multidisciplinary approach to treating problems that were outside the scope of teeth and dentistry. My mother was a myofunctional therapist trained by Daniel Garliner who saw many of our TMJ and pediatric patients.

Over the years, I also took many courses and attended many conventions, read my dad's book, and learned from other providers in fields such as physical therapy, osteopathy, chiropractic, and craniosacral therapy.

With all that exposure, I decided that I wanted to be an ear, nose, and throat (ENT) physician, or I was going to be a dentist that specialized in TMJ and sleep. I chose dentistry, but all through dental school, I knew I didn't really want to only treat teeth. I really wanted to specialize in something to do with TMJ. After graduation, I joined my father in his practice. Then, in 1989, after I had been working with him for a few years, I turned to treating the airway and addressing problems such as snoring and sleep apnea. I want to help patients get more oxygen and have more restorative or deep sleep.

I developed what is known as the AirwayCentric® Guide (ACG) System with the help of ProSomnus Sleep Technologies. The ACG System was the first day and night dental appliance solution to offer an integrated way of addressing airway issues. But that's just part of the picture. There is so much more to treating patients than just putting an appliance in the mouth.

EVERYTHING IS CONNECTED

A few years ago, I came across Complete Health Dentistry® after meeting Brad Bale, MD, and Amy Doneen, MSN, ARNP, DNP, through Gary Kadi of NextLevel Practice. That's when I realized that what I was really doing all day long was treating inflammation. I was using appliances to help people, but I was putting those appliances into a "dirty" mouth. I realized that patients had high- and moderate-risk oral pathogens that were increasing inflammation and leading them closer to a heart attack, a stroke, diabetes, or dementia.

The BaleDoneen Method® really influenced me to start looking at these oral pathogens and helping to manage them with a cardiologist or a physician that believes in the BaleDoneen Method, and now, every one of my patients undergoes bacterial testing.

That's one way we get to the source of the problem, because that's what we focus on with patients. We want to know the "why" behind their current health situation instead of just treating the symptoms. Understanding how the patient arrived at their current diagnosis in the first place—their health history, what treatments they have received from other healthcare and dental professionals—gives me a better idea of how to treat the patient.

You see, everything is connected, and when there's a problem in one area of the body, it can cause problems in other areas of the body. Some people are affected from the top down, meaning they have a problem with their jaws that causes pain in their head and neck that then travels down and affects other areas of their body. Other people are affected from the feet up—they have foot problems that travel up the body and cause problems all the way through the head. Treating the problems can take a team of specialists using an integrative approach and looking at the whole body to ensure the entire support system works together to make the body healthy.

What I bring to that team is airway. If someone comes in for treatment and reports fatigue as a symptom, we look for the source of the problem—and that means looking at more than just oral pathogens. Sleep apnea causes hypoxia; it lowers oxygen levels in the body. It also causes disturbed and fragmented sleep, depriving you of the deep, restorative sleep your brain and body need.

If the airway's closed at night, it's a tremendous source of inflammation for the entire body. Systemic inflammation leads to dysfunction of the body's cells and circulatory system. As we get more inflammation, our blood vessels lose their elasticity—leading to a host of problems—and we're keeping the sympathetic nervous system activated. Basically, your body is constantly in a state of alarm. With anti-inflammatory dentistry, we're getting rid of the high-risk oral pathogens and opening the airway. I'll talk more about all this in the chapters ahead.

What it boils down to is that, as a dentist, by identifying problems in the mouth, I am a key supporting member of a team that can address health problems everywhere in the body.

A NEW VIEW

Dentistry has become a very exciting field because of all the ways we're able to change aesthetics and so much more. Today, we're able to change growth and development, energy levels, and even cognitive levels. We now have the know-how and tools to develop the airway in children as early as two years old. Traditionally, the orthodontist never wanted to see a child until age eight or nine. But we now know that if we expand the palate enough, since the ceiling of the palate is the floor of the nose, then we can give a child a lifetime of good health. With an open airway established in childhood, that patient never suffers from sleep apnea or all the health problems that can result from it.

That includes cognitive health. That's right—we can change cognition and people's behavior just by giving them better-quality sleep. We're actually helping brain development in kids while helping with their facial development. It's a very exciting field because we can really help children and adults develop to their full potential.

Over the years, there's been a change in the understanding of whole-body health by patients as well. Today, people are more open to root-cause medicine, functional medicine, and integrative medicine. They don't want to just take a pill. They're starting to understand that there is no silver bullet and that lifestyle has a lot to do with chronic disease.

It's an entirely different focus of dentistry. We used to spend our time debating the best way to ensure that the teeth come together in the ideal bite. Today, it's all about airway—breathing trumps everything else in dentistry. If you can't breathe, it doesn't matter if you have beautiful teeth.

Let me tell you more about the different ways in which dentistry today is making an amazing difference in people's lives.

CHAPTER 2

A REVOLUTION TAKES ROOT

My patient Cara Wells was sick.

She didn't know *how* sick until it was almost too late.

On the outside, she was perfectly healthy. Cara was thirty-six, fit, and slender—she'd completed a half marathon earlier that year. She had a job she loved and two smart, rambunctious children. Cara and her husband, Ron, were high school sweethearts, still very much in love after twenty years. They had a great life.

Cara wouldn't become my patient until sometime later, after she left her old dentist and came to see me. At her first appointment, she showed me pictures of her son and daughter, telling me with tears in her eyes how close her children had come to losing their mom. As we sat in my office, I asked her to tell me her story.

"It was an ordinary morning," she began.

Cara was running late, trying to get her kids to eat scrambled eggs instead of the sugary cereals they craved. Her daughter, Alyssa, kept changing her outfit, and her son, Peter, was trying to finish his third-grade art project, which meant there were cotton balls and glue sticks all over the kitchen table. Cara was running between the bathroom and living room, trying to manage the kids and make herself presentable, when suddenly her chest felt heavy.

At first she thought she was just feeling rushed. She hadn't slept well the night before, and since Ron was away on a business trip, she'd been more stressed than usual taking care of both kids while balancing her work responsibilities. She took a couple of deep breaths, trying to make the heaviness go away.

But with every breath, the heaviness got deeper, like an anvil sitting on her chest.

As a mom, Cara was used to making the best of a bad situation. She got both her kids to school, even managing to carry in Peter's sticky art project without getting glue on her suit jacket. When she climbed back in the car, she took a deep breath. Surely now the heaviness in her chest would lessen.

But it didn't. Her chest was tighter than it had been half an hour before, so tight she knew something was wrong.

Cara called into work. "Take care of yourself, Cara," her boss said, and she thought for the hundredth time how lucky she was to have such a great boss. She called Ron, but it went straight to voice mail, so she decided to drive herself to the hospital.

When the emergency room doctor asked her why she'd come in, she said, "Chest discomfort."

The doctor examined her briefly. "Pneumonia," he said.

"But I don't even have a cough."

That didn't seem to worry him. He prescribed an antibiotic for pneumonia and sent her on her way.

"You'll feel better tomorrow," he said.

But Cara didn't feel better. The following morning, the chest pressure was even worse. It was so bad she couldn't finish making her kids breakfast—her daughter came in to find Cara doubled over the kitchen counter, a carafe clenched in her fist as coffee spilled onto the marble.

"Mom?" Alyssa said, frightened to see her mother this way. "Are you okay?"

"I'm okay," Cara said, but she didn't believe it. Something was definitely wrong.

She called her sister to take the kids to school—and then drive her straight to the ER.

This time, Cara saw a different attending physician. The new doctor examined her carefully, asking about her symptoms, medical history, and other risk factors.

The new diagnosis wasn't pneumonia. Not even close.

"It's good you came in when you did, Mrs. Wells," the doctor said. "You are having a heart attack."

At first Cara didn't believe it.

"I thought heart attacks were for elderly people," Cara told me in my office. "I was thirty-six. I'd just run a half marathon! And sure, I didn't always eat the way I knew I should. I had a soft spot for chocolate chip cookies. But I generally ate healthy, and I was hitting the gym four to five days a week."

Cara told the doctor she couldn't be having a heart attack. That it just wasn't possible.

"It's true, we don't usually see this in someone so young," the doctor said. "But you have vascular disease."

Cara was in shock. She never imagined something like this would or even *could* happen. Vascular disease was something other people had to deal with—her granddad, or her aunt Marjorie, or that big jolly guy who worked in accounting and gave himself insulin shots in the break room at lunch.

"But suddenly it wasn't a statistic or something that happened to someone else," Cara explained. "It was happening to *me*."

Her husband brought her children to the hospital that night, and they all ate vanilla pudding cups from the cafeteria and laughed and hugged each other.

"After Ron took the kids home," Cara said, "I sat in the hospital bed and sobbed. I felt so grateful to be alive, but I was also terrified. I'd always assumed I was so healthy. I didn't know what happened to get me there, in that hospital bed, recovering from a heart attack. The same question kept playing in my head: "How do I make sure this never happens again?"

I knew then what Cara didn't yet know herself—that she was on the path to complete and transformative health.

I knew something else too—the answer to her question was in her mouth.

FROM TREAT IT AND BEAT IT TO TRANSFORMATIVE HEALTH

I've spent many years studying the connection between a healthy mouth and a long, healthy life. Oral health is not tangential—though some people have spent their entire lives ingesting that lie. What's happening in your mouth is an excellent indicator of what's happening in the rest of your body, providing a holistic snapshot of your overall health.

The problem is, many of today's practitioners aren't interested in holistic snapshots. They're fixers, highly skilled at what I call "treat it and beat it." They want to treat the current symptoms so they can beat the disease. And while I'm all for beating disease, that approach leaves something to be desired.

To understand where this attitude came from—and why it persists—we need to first understand the growing pains healthcare has gone through since the dawn of time. I want to introduce you to Dr. Chip Whitney, a pioneer in the field of transformative health, whose wisdom has had a powerful influence on my own complete health practice. It was Dr. Whitney who introduced me to the three eras of health identified by Dr. Lester Breslow in the *American Journal of Public Health*.[1]

The first era started at the beginning of humankind. From the shamans and medicine men, early practitioners were literally and figuratively wandering in the dark. Health providers didn't have a lot of tools, and the tools they did have often yielded the opposite result from the ones they intended. Take, for example, the doctors who leeched sick people, believing their "bad blood" was at fault—inadvertently killing their patients, who died from loss of blood.

In the early days of human history, the focus was on battling infectious diseases. These diseases killed people in staggering numbers. The bubonic plague that swept through Europe in the fourteenth century—nicknamed the "Black Death"—killed an estimated fifty million men, women, and children, somewhere between 25 and 60 percent of the European population.

In light of statistics like that, no wonder the first era of healthcare was about survival. Infectious diseases were claiming millions of lives, so the only thing that mattered was trying to stop them through whatever means possible.

---

1 Lester Breslow, "Health Measurement in the Third Era of Health." *American Journal of Public Health* 96, no. 1 (January 2006): 17–19, https://www.ncbi.nlm.nih.gov/pmc/articles/PMC1470427/.

Now fast-forward a few hundred years. By the early 1900s, medicine had made significant advances. As public health trends improved, doctors and researchers had access to new tools and treatments. They developed antibiotics, which transformed the healthcare landscape forever.

In 1956, Elvis Presley posed publicly for his polio vaccination. This came at a time when tens of thousands of children were dying from polio, and those who weren't killed were often permanently paralyzed. Elvis's plug was highly effective; even though the vaccine had not yet been thoroughly tested, parents lined up to have their children inoculated.

Suddenly, a world that had been shrouded in darkness was exposed to the light—and the second era of healthcare began.

If the first era was about battling infectious diseases, the second era was about combating *chronic* diseases. In the latter half of the twentieth century, medicine advanced at an astonishing rate. Doctors began to identify and treat cancers. Surgery went from being a risky endeavor with terrifying instruments and a high mortality rate to a procedure that saved countless lives. Heart surgeons and brain surgeons undertook formidable challenges—and surpassed them with flying colors. Over the last fifty years, the amount of technology, medicine, and treatment options has been revolutionary.

But how does that explain people like Cara Wells? How did a seemingly healthy thirty-six-year-old woman suffer a heart attack that nearly ended her life?

The answer is simple. The second era of healthcare, as wonderful as it is, is still fundamentally flawed. The mindset of every physician in this country is "find the disease and fix it." In other words, "treat it and beat it." It is reactionary, not proactive. It treats the patient as an amalgam of symptoms and complaints, not a unique, complex human being who needs *healthcare*, not just *sick care*.

The third era of healthcare is about *mindset*. We need a new mindset among all health professions to help our patients create health, not just react to disease. The creation of health is not just about feeling okay today. It's about feeling great tomorrow—and all the tomorrows after that.

Our goal is to take a person who is not yet sick—who may not even have developed a problem—and prevent them from ever going down a path that will create an illness.

> We need a new mindset among all health professions to help our patients create health, not just react to disease.

Our main focus is simple yet powerful: *we create health.*

And who's at the cutting edge of this new third era?

We are. Your friendly neighborhood dentists.

IT'S ALL CONNECTED

I'm going to tell you something you might not want to hear.

Cara Wells could be anyone.

She could even be you.

In the human body, nothing happens in a vacuum. Everything is interconnected. But it is only now, in this third era of healthcare, that we are beginning to understand how and why.

You might be doing everything right: exercising, eating well, going in for your yearly checkups. If that's the case, more power to you. But if your dentist isn't lasering in on your oral health to look at the bigger picture, they're doing you a grave disservice, one that could mean the difference between life and death.

For years, dentistry has been associated with pain, both financial and physical. If that's the way you feel about going to see the dentist, I understand completely. Why would you willingly engage in something that only causes you pain? Only an idiot would sign up for that! I know exactly where you're coming from.

But I have good news for you. When you start thinking about dentistry in the context of complete health, it transforms from a place of pain and dread to a place of empowerment, where you, the patient, get to play an active role in your own care. Every day I partner with my patients in ways that are exciting, transformative, and even fun. Once you embrace the mouth as the gateway to complete health, great things can happen.

When I see a patient in my practice, my goal is not to drill, fill, and bill. I'm far more interested in the bigger picture of my patient's overall health.

That's why I use a process I like to call *projection diagnostics*. Projection diagnostics is a fancy term for a straightforward concept. I'm trying to project the patient's future health path based on the results of diagnostic testing technologies, such as blood and urine tests.

If a patient is on a bad health path, they can typically see right in front of them where their problems lie, and we can course correct. The trickier patients are the ones like Cara Wells, people who *seem* to be healthy, but underneath the surface, there's something more serious going on.

When Cara first came to see me, I was determined to figure out *why* she had suffered a heart attack. So I took off my white coat and donned my detective hat, ready to solve the mystery.

Cara was not at high risk for vascular disease. She was fit, young, and healthy. But I knew there must be something inflammatory going on, because heart attacks are caused by inflammation, and the inflammation that led to the heart attack had to come from somewhere.

We used the process of elimination. Cara didn't have a sprained ankle. She had no open wound. So where was the inflammation coming from?

What she *did* have was a sore tooth.

I kept digging. I sent her to an endodontist who performed a root canal. What the endodontist discovered was that the tooth was badly infected. The bacteria from the infection likely entered her bloodstream and elicited an inflammatory reaction wherever they landed, including vulnerable coronary arteries, creating the ideal conditions for a heart attack.

That's right: a tooth infection drove Cara's vascular risk. What she thought of as a minor nuisance—a sore tooth, something a couple of ibuprofens could fix—had nearly ended her life and robbed her children of their mother.

THE MOUTH IS THE GATEWAY

America is the wealthiest nation in the world, yet we are one of the unhealthiest. If that surprises you, I understand. Until I shifted my focus to complete health, I didn't know all the depressing statistics—and I certainly didn't know how to change them. But there is evidence-based science to support the oral-systemic connection.

The mouth is the gateway to the body. It has key physiological functions that make it essential to our health and well-being—we eat with our mouths, we breathe through our mouths, we have immunity through our mouths. We kiss with our mouths too, and our oral health can even determine things like social status and hirability. If your teeth are badly decayed or missing entirely, you probably aren't going to get that front-row job.

For years doctors have overlooked the connection between what happens in a person's mouth and what happens in the rest of their body. The third era of healthcare requires a seismic shift. The better we understand—and care for—our oral cavity, the better chance we have of living a long, healthy life.

In this book, we're going to examine the mouth as a gateway to overall health. When bacteria from the oral cavity enter our bloodstream and spray everywhere, our body responds with inflammation, which sparks an inflammatory cascade. This cascade can lead to cardiovascular disease, dementia, cancers, sleep apnea, obesity, diabetes, and pregnancy complications—all of which we'll talk about in depth.

For each of these diseases, we'll look at the role your oral health plays and how to identify—and treat—early warning signs. Some of the chapters include sections titled "What Can You Do about It?" This is where I'll share specific treatment options and ways to predict and prevent serious disease so that you never find yourself in a situation like Cara Wells, facing a sudden heart attack with no idea why.

I don't want you to feel scared and daunted after reading this book. I want you to feel empowered. My goal is to arm you with both the tools and strategies you need to make informed decisions about your mouth, your health, and your life.

In the pages that follow, I'll introduce you to experts and practitioners who have studied chronic disease extensively and understand the crucial role of oral health. These doctors, nurses, and researchers are paving the way for a new kind of healthcare. They have not only revolutionized the way I run *my* practice; they are leading the charge for Complete Health Dentistry around the world.

You are standing at the precipice of the third era. Together, we have the power to transform healthcare in our world, our country, and our individual lives. True "healthcare reform" isn't political. It's about treating the whole person and taking a long view, rather than sticking a bandage on as a temporary solution.

It isn't about treating and beating.

It isn't about drilling and filling.

It isn't even about dentistry.

It's about *you* and your health. I want to ensure that you are happy and healthy for many years to come.

To do that, we have to talk about the original offender: the root cause of all the diseases we'll be discussing in this book.

I'm talking about the silent assassin that nearly ended Cara Wells's life at thirty-six years old.

Inflammation.

CHAPTER 3

INFLAMMATION: THE SILENT KILLER

I want you to imagine a beautiful antique car in an auto show. The paint is candy-apple red, polished to a fine sheen. The interior is flawless. The owner took very good care of his prized possession, so there's not a spot of rust on it—not even when you pop the hood. The car has impeccable maintenance records, and all these years later, if you turn the key in the ignition, the engine still purrs.

Unfortunately, we human beings are rarely so well maintained.

Maybe you've had to face one or more diseases in your life. Maybe you haven't. But either way, you are rusting. That's just part of life on this earth. The scientific term for "rusting" is oxidation, which leads to inflammation, which leads to a host of nasty diseases that range from unpleasant to fatal.

We all live in a state of chronic inflammation. That's the basis for every single disease—cardiovascular disease, dementia, cancers, and other chronic ailments. In the last chapter, I talked about the inflammatory cascade. But since the word "inflammation" can feel esoteric and hard to quantify, I like to explain it in more concrete terms.

Let's say you're chopping vegetables in the kitchen. Your hand slips, and you nick your finger with the knife. Nothing major—no need for a trip to the emergency room—but it stings, so you hold it under the faucet for a few minutes until it stops bleeding. Then you make an impromptu tourniquet out of a paper towel and go back to chopping vegetables for dinner.

For you, the cut is over.

For your body, it's only just begun.

Your skin serves as a barrier between the inside of your body and the harmful bacteria lurking on the outside: pathogens such as bacteria, viruses, and other microorganisms. But now there's a break in the skin, providing a way for pathogens to enter your body. Once bacteria sneak in through the cut, they can infect the wound.

Now, your body doesn't throw in the towel at the first glimpse of bacteria. On the contrary—when tissue is injured or infected, the body mounts a solid defense, releasing chemicals that trigger an inflammatory response to kill the invaders.

You might be thinking, "Great, my body's a fighter!" And that's true—at least initially. Your body ignites its inflammatory response to solve the problem and resolve the cut, and for a day or two, your fingertip gets red and puffy and feels sore. A week later, once the body has fought the bacteria and won, your finger is as good as new.

But when the triggers of inflammation never stop, our natural functioning can go haywire. Sometimes, when our bodies fight back, they don't know when to stop. This is *chronic inflammation*, which drives chronic disease.

THE WAR YOU DIDN'T KNOW YOU WERE FIGHTING

Let's talk about bacteria for a moment. These are microscopic organisms, and there are a *lot* of them. The global human population is currently around 7.6 billion, and in the volume of a single nickel, you'll find 8 billion bacteria. That's right—one nickel yields more microscopic organisms than there are people on planet Earth.

There are thirteen trillion bacteria in your intestines alone—so many that I've heard doctors describe them as an organ system in and of themselves. There are good bacteria and bad bacteria. When the delicate balance of the microbiome of your intestine gets out of whack and the bad outcompetes the good, it can lead to disease.

And then there's your mouth.

As we've established, the mouth is the gateway to the body. Unfortunately for your body, your mouth hosts billions of bacteria. Your tongue, teeth, and gums are bathing in bacteria at this very moment. Think about *that* next time you kiss your spouse.

Unfortunately for you, these pathogens get along fantastically with one another, so they stick together and multiply. Eventually they form a colony, and after long enough, that colony creates a thick layer of plaque. Think of plaque like very bad houseguests—they make your life a living nightmare, then stay forever.

If you've ever been to a dentist (and I hope you have), you've heard of plaque. But it's kind of like hearing the safety instructions on an airplane; after a while, we've heard the words so many times, they no longer have any meaning.

Here's what you need to know about plaque: it spreads.

And I don't mean spreads in the way syrup oozes slowly over your pancakes. Plaque spreads like wildfire, taking over your mouth, teeth, tongue, cheeks—anywhere it can reach. If it can find an opening in your mouth that takes it directly to your bloodstream, all the better. The ravenous bacteria will happily stalk the rest of your body, wreaking havoc wherever and however they can.

But your body is wise to plaque's game. It prepares a counter-attack, waging war by firing inflammatory bullets on these foreign organisms—which in turn makes the plaque fight harder. Like any high school football team, the bacteria know the best defense is a good offense, so they launch barriers of resistance against the inflammatory attack.

In other words, there's a microscopic war raging inside you—and you have no idea.

You have a chronic inflammatory bacterial condition in your mouth. Chronic means your body never turns off the process of inflammation. It's like cutting your finger over and over and over again. The body is beleaguered by the constant assault of bacteria without an opportunity to resolve it, so the inflammatory response never powers down. What happens then?

You get sick.

THE DEADLY DANCE

As a part of his research on complete health transformation, Dr. Chip Whitney talks about three kinds of "body pollution" that lead to disease. Just like there is pollution in the air, pollution in the body drives people down certain chronic disease paths. For Dr. Whitney the three main pollutants are oxidative stress, free radicals, and—you guessed it—inflammation.

At this point you may be thinking, "I'm strong and healthy. I've never had a serious health problem or disease. Who's to say my body won't be able to fight off bacteria without causing chronic inflammation?"

In a perfect world, your body would do just that. But this isn't a perfect world. If the cause of inflammation never stops, inflammation never turns off. The reality is that our bodies get worn down over time. We rust.

Some of the root causes of body pollution are minimally under our control. Take, for example, genetics and family history. We all have genetic predispositions to certain diseases, whether we like it or not. Then there's gut dysbiosis, where once again bad bacteria begin to dominate the good bacteria and throw everything out of balance. Insulin resistance, sleep apnea, high visceral (belly) fat—these are some of the root causes of pollution, and pollution is the root cause of disease.

It's important to note here that not all diseases are alike. In the last chapter, we talked about the bubonic plague, which we now know was caused by a single bacterium. Many illnesses can be traced back to one bacterium, including those that *didn't* cause sweeping epidemics, such as strep throat or pneumonia.

What I'm talking about is not a single bacterium. I'm talking about the massive hordes of bacteria that build up in the mouth and lower intestines and are dangerous because of *quantity*, not quality. Just one of them isn't going to cause a problem, but together they drive the infection. En masse, they steal into the bloodstream, triggering inflammation that can be transmitted to other organs.

Chronic inflammation is the root cause of almost all chronic disease. But there's one root cause of inflammation we haven't touched on. I saved the best for last.

Periodontal disease.

A.k.a. gum disease.

As a dentist, I see a lot of gum disease. I have a front-row seat to inflammation in the tissues of the mouth. It starts as gingivitis, when your gums become swollen and red and may even bleed. As the disease progresses into full-blown periodontitis, the gums can pull away from the teeth, leading to bone loss and lost teeth.

Do you see how everything is connected? It all begins with bacteria, which cause periodontal disease. The pathogens trigger the body's inflammatory response, which in turn leads to inflammation in the mouth as the body tries to fight back. The mouth is the body's gateway, so the bacteria get into the bloodstream and spray everywhere, landing in the organs, the brain, and the arteries along the way, driving the same inflammation in those distant sites that is already present in the oral cavity.

And that, my friends, is a delicate, deadly dance that drives chronic disease.

THE THREE WAR ZONES

In the following chapters, we'll take a closer look at the three most worrisome diseases that result from inflammation. We'll start with cardiovascular disease, which covers heart attacks and strokes. A stroke is exactly the same as a heart attack, only it's a brain attack instead—same process, different location.

Then we'll talk about dementia. After that, we'll discuss various cancers, including colorectal, pancreatic, and esophageal. We'll also look at the interplay between inflammation and sleep apnea, obesity, diabetes, and pregnancy complications.

> There are ways to transform your health *before you ever get sick.*

Here's my promise to you: this book is not all gloom and doom. There are ways to transform your health *before you ever get sick*. That's why every chapter ends with one simple question: "What can you do about it?" For each disease, I will share treatment options and other helpful resources. I want to show you how to change the path you're on before you end up at a destination you never want to visit.

The first step is to educate ourselves. If we don't know what we're looking for, we won't know how to fight it.

I'm a dentist, so I see all kinds of things in my practice. One thing that continues to amaze me is how many of my new patients tell me their gums bleed when they brush their teeth.

"Just a little," they say. "Nothing major."

I want you to think about this for a moment. The total area of your gums is about the size of the palm of your hand. If you looked at the palm of your hand and saw an open wound, would you do something about it? Or would you continue to let it bleed?

Bleeding gums means there's an infection. Something is definitely wrong. But many people don't see it that way. They just spit a little blood and toothpaste into their bathroom sink in the morning and go on with their day.

The problem is, the mouth is only the beginning. Periodontal disease doesn't stop in your gums. Inflammation in the gums allows bacteria to spew into other parts of the body. Your organs. Your brain. Your heart.

Remember Cara Wells, the thirty-six-year-old who nearly died from a heart attack? She thought she was fine. Her risk factor profile—based on her age, gender, genetic history, and general health and fitness—appeared to be low risk. But she was harboring silent vascular disease. The inflammation from her mouth had traveled through her arteries, causing a blockage of blood flow to the heart.

Which leads me to the question we've all been dying to ask. Was there anything Cara could have done to prevent it?

STRAIGHT TO THE HEART

At the beginning of this chapter, I asked you to imagine a mint-condition antique car at an auto show. Now I want you to envision yourself at ninety years old. What do you see? Do you see a polished antique automobile with an engine that still purrs? Or do you see a rusty old mess when you pop the hood?

If you want to be healthy and happy at ninety, you need a healthy body and a healthy brain. You should be able to be as independent and active as you want to be. To get there, you need a strategy.

Most people don't have a strategy. We have plenty of strategies about our careers, finances, professional achievements, friendships, and even romantic relationships. But when we think about creating health, we tend to think in terms of losing weight, exercising, and eating well. That's it.

Those are *tools* to creating health, not strategies. At the heart of any good health strategy is identifying early disease. That's essential, because it is chronic disease that can steal life span from even the healthiest of individuals.

Identifying early disease can be challenging, especially when that disease is asymptomatic—as it usually is. Most of us do this in some form or another already; we schedule mammograms to screen for breast cancer, colonoscopies to screen for colon cancer, and so on. Lucky for us, twenty-first-century technology is rapidly evolving, increasing our ability to identify disease at an early treatable state.

The problem is that many diseases are untreatable once discovered.

So what do we do?

The answer is simple: we have to prevent the untreatable disease. We have to make the impossible possible. And the way to do that is by connecting the dots. We can prevent disease by reverse engineering our way back to the inflammation that causes it in the first place.

The best way to start, of course, is to go straight to the heart.

CHAPTER 4

THE HEART OF THE MATTER

If I asked you to tell me the number-one killer in this country, what would you say?

Car accidents?

Cancer?

The answer—which you've probably guessed from the chapter title—is heart disease.

Cardiovascular disease is the leading cause of death and disability for both men and women in the United States. Here's another statistic that will blow your mind: recent research has found that oral infections can trigger up to *50 percent or more of acute heart attacks*!

That number is staggering, and it means Cara Wells is far from unique. The current cost of cardiovascular disease to our healthcare system is about $518 billion. And guess what?

I believe it's preventable.

Prevention starts in the dentist's chair. But before we look at the link between a healthy mouth and a healthy heart, we have to understand how cardiovascular disease works—and why it's so dangerous.

OUT, DAMNED CLOT!

Cardiovascular disease is the umbrella term for a number of different issues in the body, including the following:

- Aneurysm
- Angina
- Atherosclerosis
- Cerebrovascular accident (stroke)
- Cerebrovascular disease
- Congestive heart failure
- Coronary artery disease
- Electrical malfunctions such as atrial fibrillation
- Myocardial infarction (heart attack)
- Peripheral vascular disease
- Valve diseases

In the last chapter we talked about plaque, the nightmare houseguest nobody would ever want. The buildup of plaque causes the arteries (the blood vessels supplying oxygen to the heart) to narrow, making it harder for blood to flow. If someone is harboring silent plaque in their body, and the plaque ruptures like a volcano in the inner lining of the artery, it's bad news all around. That is a heart attack. If it occurs in the carotid artery in the neck, it causes a stroke or transient ischemic attack.

Remember how our bodies are trying so hard to protect us? When plaque ruptures the wall of an artery, our body says, "We better heal that injury!" In the same way a scab forms over the wound when a kid skins their knee, your body automatically sends a clotting cascade to heal the rupture of the artery wall.

If you shiver at the word "clotting," you should. A heart attack occurs when the blood flow to a part of the heart is blocked by a blood clot. If the clot cuts off the blood flow completely, the part of the heart muscle supplied by that artery begins to die.

This event usually occurs in a small blockage. Eighty-six percent of heart attacks occur from the rupture of a plaque so small that it would not have resulted in an abnormal stress test. Some of you may remember the NBC News anchor Tim Russert. Tim had a completely normal stress test in April 2008. He died of a heart attack in June 2008. It was not that he had a bad doctor or a bad test; he just had a small plaque that did not show up on testing. A stress test is simply not an effective screening test.

In an ischemic stroke—which accounts for about 85 percent of strokes—the process is exactly the same; it just happens in a different location. The word *ischemic* comes from the Greek *iskhaimos*, or "stopping blood." If the blood clot blocks blood flow in the heart, we call it a heart attack. If it floats from the carotid artery in our neck and lands in the brain, we call it a stroke. When the blood supply to a part of the brain is shut off, brain cells die, impeding normal functions such as walking or talking.

Some of us are genetically predisposed to heart disease, and we can't change the genes we inherited. But there is one place where we can exercise a great deal of control.

You guessed it.

Our mouths.

THE MOUTH-ARTERY CONNECTION

As usual, the culprit is inflammation.

When oral bacteria enter the bloodstream and reach arteries, these arteries can incur the body's inflammatory wrath. The same inflammatory response that causes bleeding gums will occur in the walls of a vulnerable artery. Inflammation may cause the artery to rupture and then form a clot as the natural effort to heal the rupture, and as you know, that can result in a heart attack or stroke.

There's a good deal of hard science on the link between oral health and heart disease. Studies published in prominent medical journals such as *Circulation*, *Journal of the American Heart Association*, and *Lancet* have shown the connection between infection in the mouth and cerebrovascular and cardiovascular disease. Major universities and medical institutions such as the Cleveland Clinic are already changing their standards of care to incorporate the oral-systemic associations that research has uncovered.

Take, for example, the study done on 1,163 men showing the oral bacterium *Porphyromonas gingivalis* to be associated with coronary heart disease.[2] The same scientists went back and performed an even larger study of 6,950 subjects, providing serological evidence that an infection caused by major periodontal pathogens increased the risk of future stroke.[3] Several years later, the National Institutes of Health supported a third study in which researchers detected invasive periodontal pathogens at the sites of atherosclerotic disease.[4] Bacterial

2 P. J. Pussinen et al., "Antibodies to Periodontal Pathogens Are Associated with Coronary Heart Disease," *Arteriosclerosis, Thrombosis, and Vascular Biology* 23, no. 7 (July 1, 2003): 1250–1254.

3 P. J. Pussinen et al., "Antibodies to Periodontal Pathogens and Stroke Risk," *Stroke* 35, no. 9 (September 2004): 2020–2023.

4 E. V. Kozarov et al., "Human Atherosclerotic Plaque Contains Viable Invasive *Actinobacillus actinomycetemcomitans* and *Porphyromonas gingivalis*," *Arterio-*

presence in the artery wall was actually demonstrated through DNA technology.

In other words, a significant contributor to the plaque that built up in the walls of the patient's arteries had originated in his mouth!

Further investigative work needs to be performed, as is always the case with evidence-based research. But these studies—and numerous others—have established an unequivocal link. Now that we understand this important contributor to cardiovascular disease, we're able to develop novel therapies for treating it.

Of course there will always be naysayers. In a recent guest editorial to the *Journal of the American Dental Association*, Dr. Bruce L. Pihlstrom called into question the oral-systemic link, saying, "There remains a need for more convincing and higher quality evidence that oral healthcare actually has a measurable impact on specific systemic diseases before it can be claimed that attaining good oral health can prevent systemic diseases or conditions."[5]

The response from the American Academy for Oral Systemic Health (AAOSH) was swift and mighty. The AAOSH board wrote a position paper in which it called out the *Journal of the American Dental Association* for its myopic, old-school thinking and failure to see the bigger picture.

"A little over a decade ago," the paper states, "we had no idea that the complexity of periodontal disease was enough to negatively influence glycemic control or cardiovascular health. But it is a disservice to unknowing patients when practitioners neglect the mounting associations, causation, and level-A evidence that infection in the mouth significantly contributes to medical conditions such as

---

sclerosis, Thrombosis, and Vascular Biology 25, no. 3 (March 2005): 17–18.

5 B. Pihlstrom et al., "Promoting Oral Health Care Because of Its Possible Effect on Systemic Disease Is Premature and May Be Misleading," *Journal of the American Dental Association* 149, no. 6 (June 2018): 401–403.

heart attacks, stroke, Alzheimer's disease, cancers, diabetes, pre-term births, and a host of other inflammatory conditions."[6]

As my friends and colleagues at the AAOSH noted, "Change is never easy. But the evidence of a significant association between oral and systemic health is incontrovertible. We must not let the complexity of this association deter us from expanding the nature and scope of our care when it is so clearly warranted."

As Dr. Whitney points out in his 2012 editorial published in *Dentistry Today*, "There is absolutely no risk to optimal dental care and home oral hygiene ... What is the repercussion if we assume oral bacteria do not contribute to vascular disease and we are wrong? We miss the opportunity to significantly impact the lives of millions of people on the path to suffer a cardiovascular event!"

WOMEN WITH HEALTHY HEARTS

I want to introduce you to Dr. Gina Pritchard, cardiovascular nurse practitioner and the founder and director of the Prevent Clinic. For Dr. Pritchard, heart attacks and strokes are *not* an inevitable part of life. She travels and speaks as an advocate for early detection and prevention of heart disease, educating people everywhere on the importance of heart health.

We often think of breast cancer as the biggest health concern for women. Most of us know a woman who has fought it, and we see the signature pink ribbons everywhere we look. The whole month of October is dedicated to breast cancer awareness. And for good reason—one in thirty women will die of breast cancer.

---

6 J. Russo et al., "AAOSH Responds to *JADA* Editorial That Claims Promoting Oral-Systemic Connection is 'Premature and Misleading,'" *American Academy for Oral Systemic Health*, June 15, 2018, https://aaosh.org/jada-response.

It may surprise you to hear that *one in three* women will die of cardiovascular disease.

The PR campaign for detecting cardiovascular disease could learn a thing or two from breast cancer, because if heart disease had the same name recognition, thousands of lives might be saved. And yet cardiovascular disease kills more men and women than all kinds of cancer combined.

Dr. Pritchard has found that many people think of cardiovascular disease as a "man's disease," which simply isn't true. Heart attacks happen to just as many women as men, though they happen on average ten years later.

Women also have a different set of risk factors to contend with. For example, polycystic ovary syndrome (PCOS) is a hormonal disorder common among women. PCOS is a genetically driven type of insulin resistance that also increases the risk of cardiovascular disease. If you are a woman with PCOS—or if you have a wife, sister, mother, or daughter with PCOS—early screening is all the more essential.

Because women often experience different symptoms of cardiovascular disease than men, it can sometimes be harder to detect. In the months before a heart attack, a woman might be unusually fatigued—which they could just as easily chalk up to a bad night of sleep. They might also experience indigestion, weak arms, a racing heart, or anxiety. While a man might complain of gripping chest pains during a heart attack, women can have subtler, less recognizable symptoms, such as nausea; pain or discomfort in the back, stomach, jaw, or neck; and shortness of breath. Because women are often unaware these symptoms might mean a heart attack or cardiovascular disease, they ignore the signs.

"I give a female twist to the complete health workup," Dr. Pritchard says. "Not just in the dental office, but the collaborative practice model where the dental community, dental team, and the medical team are working together in an integrated approach. We want to screen, appropriately diagnose, and then either treat existing cardiovascular disease—or prevent early stage atherosclerosis from developing. We can prevent an event in the future for patients with or without existing cardiovascular disease."

Dr. Pritchard believes strongly in early-stage screening. She goes around the country championing the carotid intima-media thickness ultrasound, which is being performed in more and more dental offices—and rightly so. "I did my doctoral work on early screening," Pritchard says, "and it's something that I'm helping dentists, dental hygienists, MDs, DOs, and nurse practitioners with in offices all across the United States." She hopes to expand to other countries too, as Complete Health Dentistry goes global.

Preventing cardiovascular disease *is* possible—but you won't know how to treat it if you don't know where to look.

WHAT CAN YOU DO ABOUT IT?

Here's the good news: unlike many other chronic medical conditions, cardiovascular disease is treatable and can be reversible, even after a long history of disease.

The first step is detection. As Dr. Gina Pritchard and Dr. Chip Whitney can attest, early screening could save your life. That vital journey might begin with a trip to the dentist—as long as your dentist is an advocate and practitioner of Complete Health Dentistry.

I want to introduce you to Brad Bale, MD, and Amy Doneen, MSN, ARNP, DNP. Ten years ago, when Dr. Bale and Dr. Doneen first started working together, they began to investigate the oral-systemic link. They learned that, although there are many pathologies that drive vascular events, oral health doesn't seem to get enough attention in the medical world. The more they looked into the data and literature, the more convinced they were that the same bacteria that cause periodontal disease also cause heart attacks and ischemic strokes.

So why wasn't oral health getting enough credit? Because the medical and dental communities just did not understand. They decided to take matters into their own hands.

Together, the doctors founded the BaleDoneen Method for preventing heart attacks, strokes, and type 2 diabetes. Now they teach physicians, dentists, and other healthcare providers around the world their method for early detection and treatment.

For Dr. Bale and Dr. Doneen, a critical component of early detection and treatment is simple: go to the dentist. Get your teeth and gums evaluated regularly, and accept the recommended treatment plan when you need to—not just so you can have pretty teeth but because it might save your life.

"Periodontal disease is extremely prevalent," says Dr. Bale. "Once you're thirty years of age, there's a 50 percent chance you have it. Once you're sixty-five, there's an 80 percent chance. If you don't want to have a heart attack or stroke, you need to maintain a healthy mouth, be evaluated thoroughly for periodontal disease, and if it's present, eradicate it."[7]

Dr. Bale and Dr. Doneen are so confident in their work that they actually guarantee it. Since 2008, they have offered all patients

---

7 Brad Bale and Amy Doneen, "The Vital Importance of the Mouth-Body Connection," Oral Systemic Link, accessed April 20, 2017, http://oralsystemiclink.net/patients/profile/the-vital-importance-of-the-mouth-body-connection.

treated at their clinics—the Heart Attack & Stroke Prevention Center in Spokane, Washington, and the Heart Attack, Stroke and Diabetes Center at the Grace Clinic in Lubbock, Texas—a written guarantee stating that if the patient suffers a heart attack or stroke while under their care, the doctors will refund 100 percent of the fees paid during the year.

"We get extremely high-risk patients," says Dr. Bale, "which is fine. I like a challenging patient, and I do believe you can shut down the disease process in anybody."

Dr. Bale and Dr. Doneen have worked tirelessly to synthesize all the data and develop the BaleDoneen Method, because they truly believe that heart attacks and strokes are preventable. (You can read more about their work at baledoneen.com.)

So do I. That's why I've adopted the BaleDoneen Method in my own practice—and I have seen terrific, life-altering results.

In addition to staying on top of your periodontal care, here are some other ways to minimize your risk of having a stroke or heart attack:

- Control high blood pressure (hypertension).
- Identify inflammatory cholesterol and prediabetes early.
- Follow good oral-health maintenance practices that promote healthy gums and teeth.
- Quit tobacco use.
- Eliminate inflammatory visceral (belly) fat.
- Eat a diet rich in fruits and vegetables.
- Exercise regularly.
- Drink alcohol in moderation, if at all.

- Know your genetics.
- Establish and maintain gut health.

The following are resources that might be helpful:

- http://www.heart.org
- http://www.news-medical.net
- http://www.perio.org
- http://oralsystemiclink.net
- https://aaosh.org/
- http://www.RHSLiveWell.com

WHAT'S NEXT?

Now that we've talked about heart health, it's time to move onward and upward. Because your mouth doesn't only tell us a lot about your cardiovascular health; it also tells us all about your brain.

CHAPTER 5

DON'T FORGET

When I was growing up, we lived next door to a charming gentleman named Robert. Bob was a sweet older guy. After he retired from the company where he'd worked for twenty-five years, he and his buddies would go fishing every weekend. At night they'd grill their catch, and sometimes Bob and his wife, Yvette, would invite us over to help them eat it.

My family would gather around to hear colorful stories from Bob's time in the army or tales from the time he and Yvette lived as missionaries in Guatemala. Sometimes their grandkids would come over, and since we were all about the same age, we had a great time playing in the backyard fort. We'd happily eavesdrop on the grown-ups while devouring the fresh batch of chocolate chip cookies Yvette pulled out of the oven.

Bob was in his midsixties when he started exhibiting signs of Alzheimer's. At first it was subtle. He forgot short-term things, like where he'd parked his car at the fishing dock or what he was supposed to pick up at the grocery store. He had mood swings—nothing big at first, but Bob was a mild-mannered man, so his bursts of sudden anger caught Yvette by surprise. Soon he was experiencing a lack of spatial awareness, language difficulties, and confusion.

If you've ever watched a mind deteriorate from Alzheimer's, you know it's a heartbreaking disease. It progresses quickly, and people with advanced Alzheimer's can experience major personality changes and loss of memory, so much so that they forget their own friends and family.

Within three years of Bob's diagnosis, he couldn't recognize his grandchildren or even his own wife. As his condition worsened, Yvette could no longer provide him the level of care he required. I still remember the day they led him out of the house, moving him into an advanced memory care facility so he would be safe and well cared for.

"The hardest decision of my life," Yvette said.

If you're one of the lucky few who has never had a Bob in your life, chances are your luck won't last forever. An estimated 5.8 million Americans live with Alzheimer's disease (AD)—also known as senile dementia of the Alzheimer's type—and that number is expected to grow to *14 million* by 2050.[8]

Put another way, someone in the United States develops AD every sixty-five seconds. By midcentury, someone in the US will develop the disease every thirty-three seconds.

The face of Alzheimer's may not be what you think. Early-onset AD is becoming more prevalent, so that while the vast majority of people facing the disease are still over sixty-five, some are younger.

---

8 "Fact and Figures," Alzheimer's Association, accessed November 23, 2019, https://www.alz.org/alzheimers-dementia/facts-figures.

In 2018, approximately 200,000 individuals under age sixty-five had early-onset Alzheimer's.[9]

Many of us fear we are headed toward a future of forgetting the people we love—especially those of us who've watched friends and family members decimated by this cruel, devastating disease. I won't lie to you—the statistics aren't encouraging. According to the Alzheimer's Association, "Alzheimer's disease is the only top 10 cause of death in the United States that cannot be prevented, cured, or even slowed."[10] This is arguably the most important disease Dr. Whitney refers to when he says we must prevent the untreatable.

The *good* news is that times are changing. There are an increasing number of studies suggesting what causes it. The more we learn about AD, the better chance we have of learning how to take precautionary measures to help protect us *before* it strikes.

Scientists and researchers have made—and continue to make—exciting new discoveries in the study of AD that point to the link between it and inflammation. The field of research is still young, and more studies are needed to yield conclusive results. But the research suggests that exposure to inflammation early in life can *quadruple* one's risk of developing AD later on.

First, let's talk about what Alzheimer's is, what it isn't, and how this brutal disease has left scientists scratching their heads for a very long time.

---

9 "Fact and Figures."

10 "Facts and Figures," Alzheimer's Association, accessed July 5, 2019, https://www.alz.org/alzheimers-dementia/facts-figures.

IS ALZHEIMER'S THE SAME AS DEMENTIA?

You've probably heard "Alzheimer's disease" and "dementia" used interchangeably. The reason for this confusion may be your doctor's fault. The word *Alzheimer's* tends to evoke fear and panic, so some physicians will use the term *dementia* instead. They're not entirely wrong. Alzheimer's is one *type* of dementia. But the words are not synonymous.

According to the National Institute of Neurological Disorders and Stroke (NINDS), dementia is a group of symptoms caused by disorders that affect the brain. It is not a specific disease.

NINDS goes on to say, "People with dementia may not be able to think well enough to do normal activities like getting dressed or eating. They may lose their ability to solve problems or control their emotions. Their personalities may change. They may become agitated or see things that are not there."[11]

If you find yourself thinking, "Those symptoms sound like Alzheimer's symptoms," you would be correct. There are several types of dementia, but Alzheimer's is the most common. AD is a neurodegenerative disorder defined by the Alzheimer's Foundation of America as "a progressive, degenerative disorder that attacks the brain's nerve cells, or neurons, resulting in loss of memory, loss of thinking and language skills, and behavioral changes."

Fun fact: AD was named after a German physician, Alois Alzheimer, who first described it in 1906. Sometimes I wonder how Alois would feel if he knew his name is known the whole world over but is associated with dread and fear. Maybe an incurable disease is *not* the way you want to be remembered.

---

11 "Dementia vs Alzheimer's," Fisher Center for Alzheimer's Research Foundation, accessed July 5, 2019, http://www.alzinfo.org/understand-alzheimers/dementia/.

As more and more nerve cells die, Alzheimer's disease leads to significant brain shrinkage. And since the brain runs so many of the body's operations, when your brain powers down, you power down too.

The symptoms of Alzheimer's can vary in severity and chronology. But the overall progress of the disease is fairly predictable. AD is terminal—on average, people live eight to ten years after diagnosis, though they can sometimes live up to twenty. In the later stages, autonomic functions such as heart rate, breathing, digestion, and autoimmune response are affected.

While the disease is fatal, it's often secondary illnesses that cause death, everything from heart attacks to kidney failure to pneumonia. Advanced Alzheimer's patients are usually too frail, their immune systems too compromised, to fight off bacterial infections that a healthier person could survive.

ALZHEIMER'S AND INFLAMMATION: A STICKY BOND

There's a lot of debate about what causes Alzheimer's disease, and the various theories often get contentious. Most scientists will concede that Alzheimer's results from a combination of genetic, lifestyle, and environmental factors that affect the brain over decades.

One thing we can all agree on is that there is plaque in the brains of Alzheimer's patients. As a dentist, I obviously talk a lot about plaque. But whereas plaque in your mouth is made up of sticky deposits between your teeth, neurological plaques are abnormal clusters of protein fragments that gum up and block the functioning of brain cells. It's like what would happen if you spilled soda on your laptop; the sticky liquid would gum up the circuitry and ruin your computer. The plaque spreads through the cortex in a predictable pattern as the disease progresses.

Where the plaque comes from—and why it so viciously attacks the brain's nerve cells—remains something of a mystery. Despite the billions of dollars that have been invested to crack the case, scientists are still not certain.

"We have done absolutely nothing to change the course of the disease," says Dr. Garth Ehrlich, a professor at Drexel University College of Medicine. "Other chronic diseases we have affected, because we understand what causes them. There is nothing new you can do for an Alzheimer's patient that you couldn't do twenty years ago."[12]

Dr. Ehrlich isn't the only one who feels that the direction of Alzheimer's research needs to be rerouted. His colleague Dr. Herbert Allen, chairman of Drexel's Department of Dermatology, became fascinated by research showing a link between Alzheimer's and bacteria in the brain. He pored over the work done by Swiss researcher Dr. Judith Miklossy, who found two types of spirochetes—long, corkscrew-shaped bacteria—in the brains of more than 90 percent of Alzheimer's disease patients.[13] Her research suggested that most of these spirochetes originated from the mouth. Miklossy's paper, published in 2011, was soon corroborated by other studies that found a connection between bacteria and dementia.

In 2016, Dr. Allen conducted his own study. He and his team of scientists investigated seven postmortem brains of patients with

12 Ingeno Lauren, "Do Infections Cause Alzheimer's Disease?" Drexel University News Blog, accessed July 5, 2019, https://newsblog.drexel.edu/2016/02/10/do-infections-cause-alzheimers-disease/.

13 Judith Miklossy, "Alzheimer's Disease—a Neurospirochetosis. Analysis of the Evidence Following Koch's and Hill's Criteria," *Journal of Neuroinflammation* 8, no. 90 (August 4, 2011), https://www.ncbi.nlm.nih.gov/pubmed/21816039.

Alzheimer's disease, comparing them to ten healthy brains. The results suggested that spirochetes in the brain could be creating "biofilms," films of bacteria that are slimy, glue-like, and incredibly resistant to antibiotics.

When he published the results of his study in the *Journal of Neuroinfectious Diseases*, Allen hypothesized that "spirochetes enter the brain during a dental procedure or after a person contracts Lyme, and then spin out a protective biofilm. The body's first responders try to clear the infection, but … the immune system ends up destroying the surrounding tissue."[14]

According to Dr. Allen, the cause of Alzheimer's disease may be a body's own immune system mounting an inflammatory defense—one that could be triggered from a dental procedure or chronic inflammation of the gums.

Sound familiar?

Make no mistake—Dr. Allen's hypothesis is highly controversial. The traditional medical community loves to discredit researchers who find proof of a connection between dementia and oral health. Further research is certainly needed to confirm that spirochetal bacteria—or any bacteria—can trigger the inflammatory cascade that leads to Alzheimer's disease.

But as more research is done on the link between bacteria and Alzheimer's, I believe we'll see increasing evidence of the crucial importance of a healthy mouth. Spirochetes, the offending bacteria, are found in the oral cavity. That's a fact. And since spirochetal infection occurs years or even decades before dementia manifests, a patient could potentially prevent and eradicate Alzheimer's years

---

14 Herbert B. Allen et al., "Alzheimer's Disease: A Novel Hypothesis Integrating Spirochetes, Biofilm, and the Immune System," *Journal of Neuroinfectious Diseases* 7, no. 1 (2016).

before it begins. Remember Dr. Whitney's comment, "What if we assume oral bacteria do not contribute to disease and are wrong?" This applies to Alzheimer's disease too. We have an opportunity to prevent the untreatable.

WHAT CAN YOU DO ABOUT IT?

Since there are currently no medically sanctioned ways to prevent Alzheimer's disease, this is a tricky question. Since the research on neuroinflammation is new and growing, we're still wandering in the dark.

But there is light at the end of the tunnel, as scientists and researchers begin to illuminate the path. Dr. Dale Bredesen, a professor of neurology at the David Geffen School of Medicine at UCLA, recently launched a years-long study on ten patients with AD.[15] The results of the study, published in the journal *Aging*, were landmark, the first to suggest that memory loss in patients *may in fact be reversed.* Bredesen used a complex, thirty-six-point therapeutic program that involved comprehensive diet changes, brain stimulation, exercise, sleep optimization, specific pharmaceuticals and vitamins, and multiple additional steps that affect brain chemistry.

For me, the results of Bredesen's work are encouraging. I believe an inflammatory burden early in life, as represented by chronic periodontal disease, could have severe consequences later as a contributing factor to Alzheimer's. If the link between inflammation and Alzheimer's disease is confirmed, researchers say it would add reducing inflammatory burden to the short list of preventable risk factors for Alzheimer's disease.

---

15 Mark Wheeler, "Memory Loss Associated with Alzheimer's Reversed for First Time," UCLA Newsroom, accessed July 5, 2019, http://newsroom.ucla.edu/releases/memory-loss-associated-with-alzheimers-reversed-for-first-time.

What does this mean for you?

It means go to your dentist regularly, accept the recommended treatment plan, and do everything in your power to combat inflammation when—or better yet, *before*—it strikes.

The following are some resources that might be helpful:

- http://www.medicalnewstoday.com
- https://www.brightfocus.org/alzheimers
- https://www.alz.org/alzheimers-dementia/what-is-alzheimers/
- https://www.drbredesen.com/thebredesenprotocol

WHAT'S NEXT?

We've talked about cardiovascular health and brain health—how inflammation can lead to a heart attack and might even cause brain cells to die.

But what about other systems of the body? Does inflammation cause widespread health problems in organs like your colon or your lungs?

You bet it does. In the next chapter, I'll explain how.

CHAPTER 6

AN INFLAMED BODY IS A SICK BODY

I knew Suzanne from high school. She was a varsity cheerleader, healthy and vivacious. After graduation we went our separate ways, but since we both stayed in the area, I ran into her every few months. We'd chat and catch up about our kids' schools or what was happening in the community.

A couple of years ago, I saw Suzanne at the local coffee shop, and we decided to grab a coffee together.

"Since you're a dentist," she said, "I probably shouldn't confess this to you, but I have a tooth that's really been bothering me. I think it might be broken."

Since I'm a dentist, my response was, "You should really have that checked."

"I'm a single mom," Suzanne said. "If they tell me it's going to be $30,000, there's just no way! I don't have the time *or* the money to deal with that right now."

"But it's causing you pain?"

She nodded, a sheepish expression on her face.

I urged Suzanne to have her tooth looked at, and as we parted ways, she promised me she would go see her dentist. I told her she was welcome to come by my practice, though I understood if she'd prefer to see someone she *hadn't* gone to high school with. I even wrote down some names of colleagues I trusted.

A few weeks went by, then a few months, and suddenly a year had flown by. I assumed she'd gotten her tooth checked out and everything was fine.

The next time I saw Suzanne, she was almost unrecognizable. One-half of her face looked completely different, and her voice had changed, in part because her mouth was no longer shaped the same way. She looked like she might have suffered from a bad burn or some kind of car accident that required facial reconstruction.

Despite her drastic change in appearance, Suzanne was her same bubbly self. "I know everyone is curious what happened to my face," she said. "Do you want to hear the story?"

She told me she did go to her dentist a few weeks after we'd spoken. He sent her to a doctor, who did a biopsy immediately. Three days later, he called to give her the worst news of her life.

Suzanne had stage four oral cancer. The tumor had metastasized and spread to the lymph nodes in her neck.

The doctor gave her two options. She could go home without pursuing treatment. Because of the advanced stage of her cancer, he gave her a few months to live. Or she could do radiation. There was a chance it wouldn't work—but there was also a chance it might.

"I'm the only parent my daughter has," Suzanne said. "I told him we're doing the radiation, no question."

She accepted the treatment plan, which involved a surgery called a maxillectomy, where the doctors removed the tumor from her maxilla, or upper jaw. They also performed a neck dissection, removing the lymph nodes from her neck. At the same time the doctors transplanted the fibula, her leg bone, using it to make her a new upper jaw.

"The reason I look like this," Suzanne said, pointing to her cheek, "is because the radiation destroyed part of my face. But after the radiation was over, they started doing the reconstruction. I've had three surgeries so far, and I'm still not finished."

Considering all she'd been through, Suzanne was remarkably optimistic.

"I'm just grateful to be alive, grateful that I get to be with my daughter. But I wish I'd gone to see my dentist sooner. You were right about that. Early detection is so key, and none of us were looking for it: not me, not my dentist, not my doctor. It's so easy to screen for oral cancer! It only takes a few minutes. But there's not enough focus on preventive healthcare in this country, and I suffered because of it. I wish I'd had someone who looked at my whole health picture, you know?"

I *did* know.

Every sixty minutes, one person dies from oral cancer. That's one person every hour, twenty-four hours a day. Contrary to what many people think, it isn't relegated to people who smoke or chew tobacco; it affects people of all ages, nationalities, and walks of life. Oral cancer is one of the biggest killers in our country, but it's a silent epidemic—no one talks about it.

It broke my heart to see how much Suzanne had suffered, all because the medical professionals in her life had failed her. If she had gone to see a dentist who was attuned to her complete health, her story might have been different.

"I just want people to learn from what happened to me," she said. "If I can prevent even one person from going through what I went through, it'd be worth it."

Maybe that person is you.

THE DREADED BIG C

We all know someone who has won a battle against a cancer. We also all know someone who hasn't.

Cancer isn't choosy; it picks its victims regardless of age, race, sex, gender, and socioeconomic status. Even Steve Jobs, the man who created a veritable tech empire and had access to the best healthcare in the world, died of pancreatic cancer, proving that no amount of money or power can turn back time.

Like many of the diseases we've discussed in this book, there are varying theories about what causes cancer. Research has found a connection between some cancers and what happens in the oral cavity.

In 2015, a group of Korean scientists set out to study periodontitis, the most common chronic inflammatory condition in the mouth.[16] They investigated *Porphyromonas gingivalis*, a major pathogen of chronic periodontitis, exploring the role it plays in oral cancer.

The results of their study were exciting—and revolutionary. The researchers found that *Porphyromonas gingivalis* can indeed increase

16 Na Hee Ha et al., "Prolonged and Repetitive Exposure to *Porphyromonas gingivalis* Increases Aggressiveness of Oral Cancer Cells by Promoting Acquisition of Cancer Stem Cell Properties," *Tumor Biology* 36, no. 12 (December 2015): 9,947–9960, https://doi.org/10.1007/s13277-015-3764-9.

the aggressiveness of oral cancer cells. When it comes to cancer of the mouth, periodontitis poses a serious bacterial risk.

Oral cancer isn't the only kind of cancer that is being studied by researchers as they continue to investigate the importance of a healthy mouth. Scientists have also proposed a link between oral health and esophageal, pancreatic, and colorectal cancer.

Colon cancer is cancer of the large intestine, the lower part of your digestive system; rectal cancer is cancer of the last several inches of the colon. Together, they are referred to as colorectal. Most cases begin as small noncancerous (benign) clumps of cells called adenomatous polyps; in certain cases, some of these polyps become cancer over time.

About 140,000 people in the US are diagnosed with colorectal cancer each year, and of those, 51,000 are predicted to die from the disease.[17] It is the third most commonly diagnosed cancer and the second leading cause of cancer death.[18]

Two independent studies were recently published in the journal *Cell Host & Microbe*, one from Harvard and the other from Case Western Reserve University. In each study, scientists looked at a strain of mouth bacteria that causes gum disease to determine the role it plays in colorectal cancer. The bacteria in question was fusobacteria.

Fusobacteria starts off in the mouth and is frequently associated with gum disease. Earlier studies hadn't observed the bacteria within the actual tumors, which led researchers at Harvard to look at earlier

17 "Deaths from Colorectal Cancer," American Cancer Society, accessed November 23, 2019, https://www.cancer.org/cancer/colon-rectal-cancer/about/key-statistics.html.

18 "Statistics and Risk Factors," Colorectal Cancer Alliance, accessed November 23, 2019, https://www.ccalliance.org/colorectal-cancer-information/statistics-risk-factors.

stages of colon cancer to see if this discrepancy was merely an issue of timing.

Their hunch was correct; they found fresh evidence that fusobacteria were intimately nestled within tumors of the colon. In other words, the bacteria from the oral cavity made their way to the colon, though researchers have not yet definitively proven if the bacteria move through the blood or the gastrointestinal tract.

They didn't stop there. The Harvard researchers found that fusobacteria elevated the generation of tumors in a mutant mouse strain prone to developing intestinal cancer. Infection with these microbes attracts a particular brand of immune cell—myeloid cells—which the researchers found stimulates the inflammatory responses that can cause cancer.

Inflammation was on the prowl again, this time leading to colorectal cancer. The proof was in the colon.

BREATHE IN, BREATHE OUT

In this chapter we've talked about cancer, but there's another deadly disease that has been linked to oral health (or the lack thereof): lung disease.

Lung disease is another one of those umbrella terms with many diseases nested under it. It is technically any problem in the lungs that prevents them from working properly. Tens of millions of people suffer from lung disease in the US alone.

There are three main types of lung disease:

1. Airway diseases: These affect the tubes (airways) that carry oxygen and other gases into and out of the lungs
2. Lung-tissue diseases: These affect the structure of the lung tissue

3. Lung-circulation diseases: These affect the blood vessels in the lungs

Many lung diseases involve a combination of these three types. Take, for example, chronic obstructive pulmonary disease (COPD), one of the most common lung diseases. COPD comes in two main forms: chronic bronchitis, which involves a long-term cough with mucus, and emphysema, which involves damage to the lungs over time. Smoking, genetics, and infections—including periodontal infections—are responsible for most lung diseases.

There is a fair amount of evidence linking pneumonia to oral health. Scientists have also done a good deal of research to show that good oral hygiene and frequent professional oral healthcare reduce the progression or occurrence of respiratory diseases among high-risk elderly people living in nursing homes, especially those in intensive care units.

Similar studies have shown that lung function decreases with increasing periodontal attachment loss. In layman's terms, your lungs get worse the more the periodontal support around a tooth—the bone and tissue—has been destroyed.

All of this research lends credence to a potential association between periodontitis and chronic pulmonary diseases such as COPD.

AND THAT'S NOT ALL

In this chapter we've barely scratched the surface of the different diseases in the body that have been linked to oral health. Additional studies have pointed to a link between inflammation and kidney disease, liver disease, and numerous others.

When I see patients in my practice, these are the kinds of things I'm looking for. I often think of my friend Suzanne, who implored me to help save my patients from an experience like hers.

"I hope you encourage all your patients to focus on prevention," she told me. "I firmly believe that what happened to me *can* be avoided. But you can't find the culprit if you don't know where to look."

WHAT CAN YOU DO ABOUT IT?

As with all the diseases we've discussed in this book, there's no tried-and-true method to prevention. You can control and maintain your oral health and other aspects of your lifestyle, but of course there are some things you can't control, like your genetics.

Here's the thing—you *can* control inflammation, starting right in the dentist's chair. You *can* do everything in your power to prevent the inflammation that has been linked to cardiovascular disease; stroke; dementia and Alzheimer's; colorectal, pancreatic, and esophageal cancer; and diseases of the lungs, kidney, and liver.

Yes, additional research is needed. That's how science works. Study by study, case by case, the tide begins to turn. But the writing is on the wall. In the field of oral-systemic health, the body of evidence continues to grow. No one disputes the destructive nature of chronic inflammation. If there is anything you can do to prevent, treat, and correct it, do it. DO IT NOW.

The following are some resources that might be helpful:

- http://www.cancer.org
- http://www.emedicinehealth.com
- http://www.webmd.com

- http://www.medicaldaily.com
- http://www.mayoclinic.com
- http://www.webmd.com/lung/lung-diseases-overview

WHAT'S NEXT?

We've talked about a number of diseases that may be caused by the inflammation triggered by periodontal disease. Now we're going to change it up a bit and talk about some *root causes* of inflammation outside the mouth—including obesity, diabetes, and a condition that strikes while you're sound asleep.

That's right: the root causes of disease don't rest, even when you're trying to.

Let's talk about sleep apnea and its stealthy assault.

CHAPTER 7

THE POWER OF A GOOD NIGHT'S SLEEP

Tony was a new patient, an independent contractor who had just moved to the area. He and his wife were looking for a dentist—and they found me.

Tony was a big, jolly guy. At his first appointment, he told the hygienist: "I brush twice a day and floss every night. I'm gonna be your star patient. I don't have any problems!"

I get that a lot. On rare occasions, it's actually true. But I've learned that oftentimes, a patient either doesn't know the problems they do have, or they don't want to talk about them. They're afraid of getting slammed with a massive dental bill.

When Tony's wife, Beth, came in a few days later, she told a very different story. Her eyelids fluttered as I entered the room.

"Beth," I said, "you look tired."

"I *am* tired!" she said. "My husband, Tony, snores every night. Sometimes I make him sleep in the guest bedroom. And he tells me

I have the problem. He says my ears are too sensitive! I think I need earplugs if I'm ever going to get a full night's sleep."

It's rare that a male patient comes in and tells me he snores. Usually their wives are the ones to complain. It's not just men who are in denial. I've also had female patients complain about being too tired or waking up with headaches—with no clue they might be dealing with an airway problem.

Most of the time, they don't even know what an airway problem is.

At the Gelb Center in New York City, I specialize in treating TMJ, headaches, sleep disorders, and sleep apnea. I believe that 50 percent of the patients we dentists see in our practices on any given day may struggle with an undiagnosed airway problem. Not a sleep problem. Not a breathing problem. They have a narrowed airway—and they're paying a high price.

Over the years, I have developed razor-sharp sensibilities. Within a few minutes of examining a patient and listening to them describe their symptoms, I can often tell whether they have an airway problem. It's why I launched the Gelb Center, which now maintains two offices dedicated to AirwayCentric dentistry, oral-systemic wellness, and anti-inflammatory dentistry. Through my work, I have been able to transform countless lives, and I have developed the AirwayCentric Guide (ACG) System for dentists and healthcare providers who wish to implement AirwayCentric and Complete Health Dentistry into their practice. More on that later.

In this chapter, I want to share some of my insights with you. I believe that a clear, healthy, unobstructed airway is the hidden path to well-being.

WHAT IS SLEEP APNEA?

Many of us are tired. Day in and day out, we go through our lives in a state of chronic exhaustion. We may go to bed late and get up early. We may have to be up before our kids every morning—we frantically get them ready for school at the same time we get ourselves ready for work. As a consequence of our overscheduled, overcommitted lives, no one's getting enough sleep.

We all know that when we are tired, we're not our best self. We're more susceptible to catching a cold or—heaven forbid—being laid flat on our back with a case of the flu. But not sleeping well isn't just a minor inconvenience. It can have serious, long-term effects on your health.

> But not sleeping well isn't just a minor inconvenience. It can have serious, long-term effects on your health.

If you sleep three to four hours a night, you're going to be tired no matter what I do for you. Many of my patients dutifully get their seven to eight hours of sleep a night and still wake up heavy with fatigue. They can't figure out *why* they're so tired, and as we start to trace their symptoms back to the source, we realize something else is going on.

When you breathe, air travels down your throat through your windpipe. The narrowest part of that pathway is in the back of your throat. When you're awake, muscles keep that pathway relatively wide open. When you sleep, those muscles relax, allowing the opening to narrow. The air passing through this narrowed opening may create vibrations. These vibrations in your throat cause snoring.

Snoring is not necessarily indicative of a health issue. But for some people, the throat closes too much, and not enough air can get through to the lungs. When this happens, the brain sends an alarm to open the airway—and you are briefly roused from sleep. Many times this wakes the person sleeping next to you too.

The brain quickly reactivates the muscles that hold the throat open so air can get through again, and once all is free and clear, the brain goes back to sleep. The person lying next to you may remain awake much longer.

This disorder is called obstructive sleep apnea (OSA).

OSA is breathing interrupted by a physical block to airflow despite respiratory effort. Eighty-four percent of sleep apnea is OSA, making it the most common form. The other type of apnea, central sleep apnea (CSA), is breathing interrupted by a *lack* of respiratory effort. Complex or mixed sleep apnea is a combination of OSA and CSA.

All types of sleep apnea create abnormal pauses in breathing—or instances of abnormally low breathing—during sleep. Each pause can last from a few seconds up to whole minutes and may occur five to thirty times (or more) an hour.

Have you ever been trying to watch a movie at home, but you keep getting interrupted? Maybe your child keeps running in to ask you questions, or your internet service keeps dropping, or a colleague is bombarding you with text messages, or your dog keeps barking at people walking outside. Mine barks every time a dog is on the screen!

If you have to pause your movie five to thirty times in an hour, do you think you'll be able to hold onto the thread of the plot? I'm guessing not!

That's how it is when you have sleep apnea. Your body loses the thread of the plot—the plot being a restful night's sleep.

Symptoms of both OSA and CSA include daytime sleepiness and fatigue, snoring, restless sleep, and awakening with dry mouth or sore throat. One in four patients with OSA suffers from nighttime teeth grinding, which can wear down the teeth and destroy the enamel.

It gets worse. Researchers have revealed that people with OSA show tissue loss in brain regions that help store memory, linking OSA with memory loss. Sleep fragmentation leads to inflammation—and as we've established, inflammation can make you sick.

Despite the long list of symptoms, people who suffer from sleep apnea are rarely aware of having difficulty breathing, even upon waking. You might experience chipped teeth or reflux—little hints and clues indicating sleep apnea—but the disorder is usually recognized only by a partner or friend who has witnessed an episode. Like so many harmful diseases, you may have no idea you're sick. Sleep apnea robs you of your health and vitality—and like a midnight thief, it does it while you sleep.

So far in this book, we've talked about how inflammation is a key player—the central villain, you might say—in oral-systemic health. We've seen how it can drive cardiovascular disease, dementia, and cancer, and we know that bacteria in the gums and mouth can trigger an inflammatory cascade.

But there is an *additional* cause. I believe that airway and sleep disorders are the most prominent cause of systemic inflammation, as well as oxidative stress, endothelial dysfunction, and sympathetic overload. This is why I have dedicated my life's work to helping patients open their airways. If I can increase oxygenation to allow deep sleep, I can improve cardiovascular disease, cerebrovascular disease, diabetes, and even dementia and Alzheimer's disease. Oxygen can also help eradicate the microorganisms that exist in the mouth.

I refer to those microorganisms as *bad bugs*. It is not by coincidence that the bad bugs in our mouths are anaerobic, meaning they thrive in low-oxygen environments.

What that means is when we open the airway and increase systemic oxygen, it helps to reduce oral bacteria from the inside out, lowering inflammation and reversing chronic disease and dementia.

DON'T LET THE BAD BUGS BITE

We often think of sleep apnea as a disorder that afflicts adults, particularly those who are older and overweight.

It's true that people with low muscle tone and soft tissue around the airway are at a heightened risk for OSA. Common indicators include obesity, a body mass index greater than thirty, large neck (sixteen inches for women and seventeen inches for men), enlarged tonsils, a large tongue, morning headaches, irritability, mood swings, depression, learning and memory difficulties, and sexual dysfunction. Risk of OSA rises with an increase in body weight, active smoking, and age. Diabetics or borderline diabetics are up to three times more likely to have it.

Opportunities for prevention are available far earlier than we might think. By age three or four, kids can already be dealing with allergies that negatively affect their breathing or other factors that make them mouth breathers. They might snore, which we think is cute.

But it's not cute. For kids, having even one event an hour, one moment when their sleep is interrupted, can have a devastating effect. Interrupted sleep can affect the normal development of the prefrontal cortex, and then suddenly your child might get diagnosed with attention deficit hyperactivity disorder, or other disorders, which might have been prevented by ensuring uninterrupted, healthful sleep.

If, on the other hand, the prefrontal cortex develops the way it's supposed to, it yields positive neurobehavioral and neurocognitive results. This will affect the hippocampus, the brain center of emotion, memory, and the autonomic nervous system. A healthy prefrontal cortex can make your children far less susceptible to dementia and cognitive impairment later in life. It can even decrease the risk of anxiety and depression.

You wouldn't believe how many patients come to my practice with anxiety—and since many of them see me more often than their general practitioner, I'm the one they talk to about it. I have achieved incredible results with my patients when it comes to anxiety. I can get rid of anxiety by 50 percent within two weeks, just by taking the airway that's being pinched and opening it up.

If you're anxious or depressed, you should always speak to a psychologist or psychiatrist. But unblocking the airway could be another important tool in your tool kit when it comes to combating mental illness, including drug-resistant anxiety and depression.

Good sleep habits and preventive measures can make a crucial difference to the well-being of your children, both now and in the future. Sleep is when the brain recharges. Human growth hormone gets released at night, which is pivotal as your child grows and develops.

I believe you can prevent your kids from ever getting sleep apnea. And since men are more likely to suffer from sleep apnea than women at a three-to-one ratio, just think of the positive effect this will have on your child's future relationships. Your sons will never become snorers like Tony, and your daughters will never become like poor Beth, married to a man she has to exile to the guest room just to get a good night's sleep!

WHAT CAN YOU DO ABOUT IT?

The current and developing research on sleep apnea is very hopeful. Treatment of OSA with continuous positive airway pressure and oral devices—more on those in a moment—improves levels of inflammatory markers. This is significant, considering atherosclerosis (the disease of the arteries we discussed in chapter 4) is an inflammatory disease. OSA may be the link between atherosclerosis and periodontal disease that the dental community has been so interested in, since the association between these two conditions has been supported by evidence-based research.

I have enjoyed phenomenal success in my practice. I and my team have developed a personalized care plan involving treatment of periodontal disease, laser periodontal therapy, and tray delivery system. This customized oral-hygiene plan also helps disrupt the colonization of bacteria and expose the hiding places of the bad bugs. My team of sleep experts monitors blood markers for inflammation, keeping track of how well they are doing to bring systemic inflammation down to ideal levels to keep patients at their healthiest.

At the heart of my work is the ACG System, the first fully integrated day and night oral appliance approach to solving airway issues by integrating treatment of airway and sleep for patients with TMJ. The system includes six appliances that complement the traditional ProSomnus [IA] platform, including the Day and the Night products.

The ACG Day is a lower milled repositioning device that covers the canines and establishes canine guidance while opening the airway during the day. It involves no clasps and is thinner lingually, allowing better speech—essential for a daytime appliance. It helps balance the nervous system and reduces pain while opening the airway, focusing on improving performance and energy levels while decreasing these symptoms.

The ACG Night appliance is an antiretrusion appliance with either the same repositioning bite as the ACG Day or a slightly increased vertical and protrusive bite. The anterior guide ramp prevents the jaw from retruding. These appliances stop the lower jaw from dropping back at night, preventing a collapse of the airway during sleep. The main focus of the night appliances is to alleviate OSA and snoring and to improve oxygenation, promoting more restorative sleep.

These are not your average oral appliances. While traditional night guards may prevent wear of the teeth, they may or may not improve TMJ and clenching—and many actually *worsen* sleep-related breathing disorders and snoring. I call these ACG System appliances the "Nightguards 2.0." They won't close the airway and can alleviate clicking and locking, headaches, and neck pain. You may awaken more refreshed and with better focus and memory. And of course, there are huge, long-term benefits in preventing cardiovascular disease and dementia.

At the end of the day, what if all we really need is a good night's sleep?

The following are some resources that might be helpful:

- https://www.drmichaelgelb.com/nightguard-2-0/
- https://www.drmichaelgelb.com/acg-system/
- http://www.sleepfoundation.org
- http://www.mayoclinic.com
- http://www.chestnet.org

- http://www.perioimplantadvisory.com

WHAT'S NEXT?

In the next chapter, we will discuss a condition in which a little extra weight is not only normal—it's exactly what you want. You'll also learn about how obesity and diabetes can be complicating factors for disease by aiding and abetting inflammation in the body.

If you want to know how periodontal disease can lead to pregnancy complications and preterm birth, read on.

CHAPTER 8

BABIES, BELLIES, AND BLOOD SUGAR

When Carolina and her husband, Sam, first became my patients, they wanted more than anything to have a baby. She was thirty-nine and he was forty-two, and they'd been trying to conceive for some time.

Carolina was one of those people who could make friends with anyone. She bonded quickly with my hygienist, who was also trying to get pregnant. They hit it off right away.

"We've been doing fertility treatments for the past two years," Carolina told her, "and I just don't think it's going to happen. I've always wanted to be a mother, and the thought of not being able to give Sam a son or daughter breaks my heart."

As my hygienist examined Carolina's mouth, Carolina became clearly uncomfortable. The prognosis wasn't good. When asked, she said her gums bled regularly when she flossed. Carolina had high levels of bacteria in her mouth.

When we laid out a plan to get Carolina back on the path to oral health, she accepted the treatment plan without hesitation.

"Absolutely," she said. "If it means helping us improve our chances to get pregnant, we'll do whatever it takes."

Six months later, Carolina told me about when she knew she was pregnant. She woke up and noticed her breasts were more tender than usual. For the next few days, she found herself urinating more frequently, and she was bone tired in a way she'd never felt before. Then she missed her period.

Carolina tried desperately not to get her hopes up. But she was trembling when she took the at-home pregnancy test. That evening, when Sam came home from work, she couldn't wait to tell him.

"It felt like a miracle," Carolina told me. "We knew God had answered our prayers."

I like telling this story, not only because it ends as a "happily ever after" but because it demonstrates the importance of understanding the oral-systemic health connection. We were able to heal the inflammation and infection in Carolina's mouth, helping pave the way for a healthy pregnancy. Nine months later, she and Sam welcomed Sam Jr.

There are other stories that don't end so happily. Women who do not maintain a healthy mouth during pregnancy can suffer severe and heartbreaking consequences. Though the science is still evolving, studies have suggested a link between inflammation and pregnancy complications such as preterm labor, preeclampsia (rise in blood pressure), and even stillbirth.

This is not something any pregnant couple should have to endure—which is why we need to talk about it, to ensure it never happens to you.

BACTERIA IS BAD FOR YOUR BABY

Here's a statistic that may surprise you: according to the World Health Organization, the US ranks sixth among the top ten countries for premature births.[19] Twelve percent—more than one in nine of all births—are preterm. That's half a million babies each year.

Dr. Yiping Han is a researcher at the College of Dental Medicine at Columbia University. Her focus is on oral microbiology; she studies how oral bacteria cause infections in the mouth and elsewhere in the body.

In 1996, a study was published providing the first evidence that women with periodontitis had a tendency to deliver premature and low-birth-weight babies. Since then, there have been a number of supporting epidemiological studies. In a paper published in the *Journal of Dental Research*, Dr. Han dug deep into the existing research. She concluded that "evidence is accumulating that oral bacteria may translocate directly into the pregnant uterus, causing localized inflammation and adverse pregnancy outcomes."[20]

In layman's terms, this means that if bacteria from the mouth sneak into the blood circulation, they spray everywhere. Sound familiar? Some make their way into the uterus, where they can lead to infection, causing the sack of fluid to break prematurely, preterm labor, and—in worst-case scenarios—stillbirth.

To put it bluntly, it could kill the baby.

The findings from Dr. Han's studies are significant because they challenge the existing paradigm in the medical community. When

---

19 Partnership for Maternal, Newborn & Child Health, "Born Too Soon: The Global Action Report on Preterm Birth," news release, May 2, 2012, http://www.who.int/pmnch/media/news/2012/preterm_birth_report/en/index3.html.

20 Yiping Han, "Oral Health and Adverse Pregnancy Outcomes—What's Next?" *Journal of Dental Research* 90, no. 3 (March 2011):289–293, https://www.ncbi.nlm.nih.gov/pubmed/21041548.

doctors find an intrauterine infection, it's usually believed to originate in the vaginal tract. But Dr. Han's studies show that the bacteria may *not* come from the vaginal tract—and could very well come from the mouth through the bloodstream. In fact, oral bacteria might account for anywhere between 10 and 30 percent of these infections.

Needless to say, the cost of bacteria invading a pregnant woman's uterus is incredibly high—physically, financially, and emotionally. When a family loses a baby, it can be crushing. Grieving parents often wonder, "Was this my fault? What did I do wrong?" It breaks my heart to hear that question. I would love to prevent this kind of loss for as many parents as possible. It's a mission I strongly believe in—and one of the reasons I wanted to write this book.

Then there are couples like Carolina and Sam, who had a long, hard road to pregnancy in the first place. This infection can also infect the uterus in women who are not yet pregnant. It can make it exceedingly difficult to conceive in the first place or can kill the baby before it's even a known pregnancy; most miscarriages happen in the first twelve weeks.[21]

Compounding the problem in some, there is strong science to support the thesis that women on fertility treatments may have trouble getting pregnant because the extra hormones given to stimulate fertility are absorbed into the estrogen receptors in their gums. If there is already bacterial infection present, the hormones can exacerbate it.

Intuitively, the oral-systemic connection makes sense. An infected uterus is a high-risk place for a tiny human to develop. A healthy mouth contributes to an environment that can allow for a healthy, successful pregnancy.

---

21 "What Is a Miscarriage?" WebMD, accessed July 5, 2019, https://www.webmd.com/baby/understanding-miscarriage-basics#1.

WHAT CAN YOU DO ABOUT IT?

We've all heard about strange pregnancy cravings, whether we've had them ourselves, known women who have had them, or seen them on TV. We joke about a mom-to-be needing her sardines and ice cream, but at the end of the day, she would do well to ditch the ice cream. The more frequently you give into the craving for sugary snacks, the greater the chance of developing tooth decay. Studies have shown that the bacteria responsible for tooth decay pass from the mother to the child in utero. Not something you want your baby to inherit!

There are other aspects of pregnancy that make it more difficult to maintain good oral hygiene. For example, pregnant women with acid reflux are at a greater risk of tooth erosion and periodontal problems, as the acid begins to thin and wear away the enamel—the protective coating of the teeth—leaving them weakened. If you are experiencing acid reflux, you should talk to your dentist about ways to combat these negative effects.

Increasingly, insurance companies are recognizing the value of healthy gums during pregnancy and are encouraging hygiene cleanings—and so do I.

The following are some resources that might be helpful regarding pregnancy:

- http://www.americanpregnancy.org
- http://www.webmd.com/oral-health/dental-care-pregnancy
- http://www.disabled-world.com
- http://www.whattoexpect.com
- https://www.perio.org/consumer

Now let's talk about when you're carrying extra weight that's *not* a bun in the oven.

OBESITY, DIABETES, AND PERIODONTAL DISEASE: A VICIOUS CYCLE

We've touched briefly on obesity and diabetes as complicating factors of other diseases, but I wanted to add a few words here. Obesity is a medical condition in which excess body fat has accumulated to the extent that it may have an adverse effect on health. More than one-third of US adults are obese. It is well known that obesity can increase the likelihood of sleep apnea, heart disease, type 2 diabetes, and certain types of cancer.

In a study published in the *Journal of Periodontology*, obese individuals between the ages of eighteen and thirty-four were found to have a rate of periodontal disease *76 percent higher* than individuals with a healthy weight.[22] Obese patients have more tooth decay and more missing teeth. Since diet is partly to blame, I always encourage my obese patients to avoid sugary drinks, limit snacking, and eat a well-balanced diet. Bacteria love sugar as much as the rest of us, and when they feed on the sugars in food, they make acids. Over time, these acids destroy enamel, resulting in tooth decay.

Obesity and diabetes are often linked, insofar as obese men and women—especially those with belly fat—are at a higher risk for type 2 diabetes. And to further connect the dots, gum disease is considered the sixth complication of diabetes. Patients with uncontrolled type 2 diabetes are at a much higher risk for gum disease.

---

22 M. S. Al–Zahrani, N. F. Bissada, and E. A. Borawskit, "Obesity and Periodontal Disease in Young, Middle-Aged and Older Adults," *Journal of Periodontology* 74, no. 5 (May 2003): 610–615.

It's a vicious cycle because severe periodontal disease can increase blood sugar—and poor sugar control is what causes diabetes. Diabetes is a condition in which a person has high blood sugar (glucose). This occurs either because the insulin production is inadequate or because the body's cells do not respond to insulin or both.

Insulin's job is to pull glucose out of the blood and give it to tissues that need it. If you have an active periodontal infection, your blood sugar level stays elevated, because when you have an infection of any kind in your body, it stimulates your liver to release sugar in an effort to fight off the infection.

Additionally, studies have shown that diabetics have a decreased ability to fight infections, including infection in the gums. This increases the bacterial load in the mouth, making gum inflammation worse. Together, these increase the likelihood that bacteria enter the bloodstream to drive disease at distant sites. We've all heard the nightmare stories of diabetics who have had to amputate toes or even limbs.

Don't let this happen to you.

By now you probably see the circular nature of these conditions: diabetes can lead to periodontal disease, and periodontal disease can cause—and exacerbate—diabetes.

Researchers recently performed a study premised on the question, "Which comes first, diabetes or periodontal disease?"

They followed the test subjects for years. One in particular stood out, a happy, healthy thirty-five-year-old woman with neither periodontal disease nor diabetes when the study began. About three-and-a-half years later, she developed severe periodontal disease. So much bone was lost that her teeth actually migrated, and some of her back teeth were at risk of falling out.

What the researchers found was that, in the time between the two visits, this woman had also developed diabetes. If a patient has diabetes and also has periodontal disease, the periodontal disease makes diabetes worse—and vice versa.

This is a perfect example of the interaction between the mouth and the body. The oral-systemic link can work in *both* directions, a deleterious dance of cause and effect.

The following are some resources that might be helpful regarding obesity and diabetes:

- http://www.obesityaction.org
- http://www.cdc.gov/obesity/data/adult.html
- www.medicalnewstoday.com/info/diabetes
- https://www.perio.org/consumer/gum-disease-and-diabetes.htm

WHAT'S NEXT?

We've talked about the relationship between inflammation and cardiovascular disease, dementia, cancers, sleep apnea, pregnancy complications, obesity, and diabetes.

We've talked about the vast and far-reaching consequences of periodontal disease on your health, happiness, and life.

But what are the broader implications of the oral-systemic link? As we move into a third era of healthcare, how do our choices affect our cities, our country, and our world?

CHAPTER 9

THE COST OF DOING NOTHING IS TOO GREAT

I'm proud to be an American. I think we live in the greatest country in the world.

But to be honest with you, I believe we have some work to do when it comes to keeping people healthy, happy, and free to live long, independent lives. Our current healthcare system isn't about "health" at all—and that needs to change. We have a *sick-care* system.

Today's medical costs can be crushing. They certainly aren't competitive with other countries—healthcare in the United States is *twice* as expensive as in Europe and four times as expensive as in Mexico, Japan, India, and China. Major companies have figured this out, which is why they've

Our current health-care system isn't about "health" at all—and that needs to change. We have a *sick-care* system.

created incentive programs and wellness initiatives to encourage preventive care.

Our country has hit a pivotal inflection point. Healthcare has to become less expensive, and in my mind, the only way to accomplish that is to better maintain good health—and that starts with taking better care of our mouths.

In 2014, a landmark paper was published in the *American Journal of Preventive Medicine.*[23] In the study—the first of its kind—researchers from the University of Pennsylvania conducted a comprehensive, five-year project in which they evaluated the claims of nearly 1.7 million patients covered by Highmark Health and United Concordia Dental. The researchers were looking specifically at patients with chronic medical conditions and also pregnant women.

What they discovered was remarkable. Out of almost 1.7 million patients, 338,891 people who suffered from a chronic medical condition had also been diagnosed with periodontal disease. That's a solid 20 percent.

The researchers didn't stop there. They drilled down into the dollars and cents of the research, lasering in on patients who were actually *treated* for their gum disease. They found the annual financial savings to be impressive. People with coronary artery disease saved on average $1,090 yearly on their annual medical costs. Diabetics saved an average of $2,840 yearly. People who had suffered from a stroke saved a whopping $5,681. Women who were pregnant saved $2,433.

In my opinion, the savings in this study was significantly underestimated. The Centers for Disease Control and Prevention estimates that 47.2 percent—nearly *half of American adults*—have periodontal

23 "The Mouth: The Missing Piece to Overall Wellness and Lower Medical Costs," United Concordia Dental, accessed July 5, 2019, https://www.unitedconcordia.com/docs/united%20concordia%20oral%20health%20whitepaper.pdf.

disease.[24] The fact that only 20 percent of the study participants had periodontal disease noted in their dental records proves the condition is severely underdiagnosed. If all those with periodontal disease had been identified and treated, the savings would have been much, much higher.

Thousands of dollars saved, simply by getting a healthier mouth.

HAVING A HEALTHY MOUTH IS SOMETHING TO BE PROUD OF

If the mouth is the gateway to complete health, then it follows that keeping our mouths healthy is the gateway to a stronger, healthier America.

But change doesn't happen on its own. There is a specially trained group of men and women in this country who will have to step forward and offer preventive care if we want to kick-start the revolution.

I'm one of them. Your friendly neighborhood dentist.

Or if you prefer something a little fancier, "oral-systemic specialist."

I'm guessing that, before you read this book, dentists would *not* have been the first professionals to come to mind when you imagined solving our nation's health problems. But if you think about it, we dentists are in the *ideal* position to make a tremendous influence on our healthcare system.

Generally, people are already in the habit of visiting the dentist every six months—way more often than the average American visits their primary-care physician. And as you now understand better, pre-

24 P. I. Eke et al., "Prevalence of Periodontitis in Adults in the United States: 2009 and 2010," Journal of Dental Research 91, no. 10 (August 30, 2012): 914–920, http://journals.sagepub.com/doi/abs/10.1177/0022034512457373.

venting disease is significantly less costly than trying to cure people once they have it. Considering the 162 diseases with early warning signs that can be detected in the mouth, we dentists may in fact be the *perfect* health professional to prevent and reverse disease.

> Generally, people are already in the habit of visiting the dentist every six months—way more often than the average American visits their primary-care physician.

In other words, the system is already set up for the solution.

There has to be a contextual shift in how we think about the mouth. As Dr. Whitney says, we need to move into the third era of dentistry. Many dentists are still trapped in the old-school way of thinking. They subscribe to the "drill, fill, bill" mentality, or like so many physicians today, "treat it and beat it." We're trained to find the chief complaint and fix it. But that's a reactive care dentist. That's not the person who's going to be leading the revolution.

The times we're living in call for a new kind of dentistry—and to go with it, a new kind of dental team.

When we graduated from dental school, we were taught to be problem solvers. In this new context of complete health, we understand that the body affects the mouth and the mouth affects the body.

For me personally, this shift in mindset has allowed me to look at the whole patient. When I started asking people about their general medical history and their family history, I found that many of them hadn't been to see their physician for a checkup in years. That gave me the opportunity to engage in conversations with them about everything from smoking to exercise to getting that appointment with their primary-care physician to get a long-overdue physical.

When a patient comes into my practice, I don't just ask, "Is anything bothering you?" with the intent of fixing it and sending them on their merry way. I look at their health from a wider scope. When I'm treating their periodontal disease, I'm also looking for signs and symptoms of other diseases or conditions. I encourage them to go see their general practitioner to discuss the concerns we raised in the dental office.

I treat the whole person, not just the mouth. My patients see me and my team as more than just a dentist office. We care about their total body health and well-being.

Am I trying to replace physicians? Not at all. I want to *partner* with my fellow medical professionals. If the mouth is the first line of defense, that means I have a lot of responsibility to keep you healthy. I have valuable information about your health that I can share with your primary-care physician or other doctors—and I don't take that responsibility lightly. Neither do my hygienists, who are critical to providing the best care we can offer.

We are assuming our needed role in the integrated model of healthcare. When I think of the future of our country as Complete Health Dentistry takes root, I have a very clear vision. I imagine the full spectrum of healthcare practitioners coming together to provide you with the very best in holistic, integrated care. I imagine physicians understanding and embracing the importance of the oral cavity as a powerful gateway to complete health, not a separate island cut off from the rest of our body.

I imagine a world in which the public government, insurance carriers, physicians, dentists, hygienists, pharmacists, dieticians, and all health professionals understand dentistry as the first line of defense against sickness and debilitating disease.

I imagine patients who are excited to assume ownership of their own health, taking proactive and preventive measures to ensure they live a long, healthy life.

That's the reason our office practices Complete Health Dentistry. I believe dentists can change the world.

But I can't do it alone. To turn the tide as we move boldly into the third era of healthcare, there's one more person who plays a pivotal role.

You.

CHAPTER 10

NOW YOU KNOW—NOW'S THE TIME

Our focus is completely different at my practices, the Gelb Center of NYC and the Gelb Center of White Plains. Because of the tens of thousands of people that I've treated, I know what's possible when you walk in the door. I know when we begin your evaluation where you can be six months or a year from now.

We start by looking at what's happening with your function, dysfunction, and imbalances during the day; then we look at what's happening with you at night. Our goal is to address issues with your musculoskeletal and neuropathic systems to help you get the most oxygen and the deepest, most restorative sleep.

That's how we help you experience changes that you would think were impossible. As I mentioned, we want to get to the source of the problems, and that starts with the initial evaluation, an hour-and-a-half visit where we gather your history and discuss your issues, take imaging, and then develop a timeline that includes the treatments to help you go from point A to Z, with Z being your pain-free, best self.

It's all about managing habits, and that boils down to mindfulness. By teaching cognitive behavioral relaxation techniques and other ways to manage the neck, posture, cervical spine dysfunction, and jaw issues throughout the day, the body goes through a transformative process over a few months' time. Then, it's just a matter of coming back in to my practice for periodic tune-ups, if needed.

IT TAKES A TEAM

I am so committed to improving airway function that I cofounded with my associate, Howard Hindin, DDS, two organizations focused on the subject: the Foundation for Airway Health and the American Academy of Physiological Medicine and Dentistry (AAPMD).

The Foundation for Airway Health is a patient-centered group that started Global O2 Day, which is a day of awareness for airway health. The organization's website, airwayhealth.org, contains information for parents and caregivers, teachers, grandparents, or anyone who knows a child, teen, or adult with an airway issue.

The AAPMD provides members with the tools and information to help them recognize the importance of the airway anatomy and physiology on sleep, development and health, and performance and function.

Part of the goal of both organizations is to promote a more collaborative effort between healthcare providers in addressing the issues that affect the airway. Traditionally, dentistry and orthodontics never really addressed the airway. In fact, historically, some dental treatments have actually worked in reverse of what we know today, promoting closure of the airway instead of opening it. Even today, too often the night guards that are prescribed do not keep the airway open. The perfect night guard that we were all taught how to create in dental school decades ago may actually be doing more harm than good. The older designs and technologies may protect teeth from being worn down from grinding, but they may worsen sleep apnea because they create height in the mouth instead of bringing the lower jaw forward.

Times have changed, and so have the treatments and technologies that we are able to use today to treat patients.

What's also changed is that getting the ultimate in care today means finding a collaborative team—the team approach will really do you the most good. To get the best results, you need a team of professionals who know how to treat TMJ, sleep, and airway—for people at every age of life—from two to ninety-two. We know that even very early on, at two or three days old, we can clip a child's frenulum so that they can breastfeed and more fully develop their mouth and swallowing functions. By starting at or even before birth (by addressing the mother's oral and overall health), we're able to help people live healthier lives and prevent problems of old age such as dementia and Alzheimer's. When it comes to airway, it's really a birth-to-death situation—the airway plays a role from the second we come out of the womb until we die.

The integrated collaborative team may also include pediatric dentists, orthodontists, prosthodontists, ENTs, and pediatric ENTs. It may include physical therapists, chiropractors, and myofunctional therapists. And it may include specialists in functional and integrative medicine that understand the BaleDoneen Method and the recode protocol. Together, we work to help patients get back to where their body can thrive.

Using a team is a more sophisticated approach that augments what we do in my office to help address treatment cognitively, behaviorally, and functionally—all the ways that you need to live your best life.

MY PROMISES TO YOU

Now that you know more about Complete Health Dentistry, it's time to reach out for an evaluation. If you choose me and my team for that evaluation and diagnosis, and that leads to treatment, here are my promises to you:

- Promise 1: You can wake up refreshed.
- Promise 2: You can have a night guard that keeps you from snoring or waking up with a headache.
- Promise 3: You can have a night guard that prevents you from wearing down your teeth and that alleviates the clicking, popping, and locking of your jaws.
- Promise 4: You can have a night guard that actually opens your airway instead of closing it.
- Promise 5: You can get rid of panic attacks and anxiety.
- Promise 6: You might be able to get off some of your medications.
- Promise 7: Your life will be dramatically transformed.

While the prospect of inflammation and autoimmune disease may be scary, it's important you get any symptoms checked out—

particularly if you suspect an airway sleep disorder, as the Airway-Centric treatment may change your life.

If you're waking up breathless at night, if you're waking in the mornings with headaches and pain, if you're so fatigued you're just trying to make it through the day, your airway may be to blame. But if we fix the underlying mechanism of your sleep breathing disorder, you'll be able to breathe easier and get a better, more refreshed sleep.

Reach out today for an evaluation to see whether your airway is causing you to have fragmented and disrupted sleep. Visit www.drmichaelgelb.com or give us a call at 212-752-1662.

NOTES

Breslow, Dr. Lester, "*Health Measurement in the Third Era of Health.*" Am J Public Health. 2006 January; 96(1): 17–19.

Pussinen PJ, Jousilahti P, Alfthan G, Palosuo T, Asikainen S, Salomaa V. "*Antibodies to periodontal pathogens are associated with coronary heart disease*". Arterioscler Thromb Vasc Biol. 2003; 23: 1250–1254

Pussinen PJ, Alfthan G, Rissanen H, Reunanen A, Asikainen S, Knekt P. "*Antibodies to periodontal pathogens and stroke risk.*" Stroke. 2004; 35: 2020–2023

Kozarov EV, Dorn BR, Shelburne CE, Dunn WA, Progulske-Fox A. "*Human Atherosclerotic Plaque Contains Viable Invasive Actinobacillus actinomycetemcomitans and Porphyromonas gingivalis.*" Arteriosclerosis, Thrombosis, and Vascular Biology. 2005;25:e17-e18.

Bale, Dr. Brad and Doneen, Dr. Amy, "*The Vital Importance of the Mouth-Body Connection.*" http://oralsystemiclink.net/patients/profile/the-vital-importance-of-the-mouth-body-connection: April 20, 2017.

https://www.alz.org/alzheimers-dementia/facts-figures

http://www.alzinfo.org/understand-alzheimers/dementia/

https://newsblogdrexeledu/2016/02/10do-infections-causeazheimers-disease/

Miklossy, Judith. Neuroinflammation. 2011 Aug 4;8:90. doi: 10.1186/1742-2094-8-90. https://www.ncbi.nlm.nih.gov/pubmed/21816039

Allen et al., "*Alzheimer's Disease: A Novel Hypothesis Integrating Spirochetes, Biofilm, and the Immune System.*" J Neuroinfectious Diseases 2016, 7:1. http://dx.doi.org/10.4172/2314-7326.1000200.

Wheeler, Mark. "*Memory loss associated with Alzheimer's reversed for first time.*" October 2, 2014. http://newsroom.ucla.edu/releases/memory-loss-associated-with-alzheimers-reversed-for-first-time

Ha, N.H., Woo, B.H., Kim, D.J. et al. Tumor Biol. (2015) 36: 9947. https://doi.org/10.1007/s13277-015-3764-9

http://www.who.int/pmnch/media/news/2012/preterm_birth_report/en/index3.html

Han, Yiping. "*Oral health and adverse pregnancy outcomes—what's next?*" J Dent Res. 2011 Mar;90(3):289-93. doi: 10.1177/0022034510381905. Epub 2010 Nov 1.

https://www.webmd.com/baby/understanding-miscarriage-basics#1

Al–Zahrani MS, Bissada NF, Borawskit EA. *Obesity and periodontal disease in young, middle aged and older adults.* J Periodontol. 2003;74:610–5

https://www.unitedconcordia.com/docs/united%20concordia%20oral%20health%20whitepaper.pdf

P.I. Eke, B.A. Dye, L. Wei, G.O. Thornto-Evans, R.J. Genco. "*Prevalence of Periodontitis in Adults in the United States: 2009 and 2010.*" Volume: 91 issue: 10, page(s): 914-920. Article first published online: August 30, 2012; Issue published: October 1, 2012. http://journals.sagepub.com/doi/abs/10.1177/0022034512457373.

www.ingramcontent.com/pod-product-compliance
Lightning Source LLC
LaVergne TN
LVHW022304200926
848481LV00004B/1219